NOT DEAD YET

World Triathlon Champions 75+ Offer Tips for Thriving & Flourishing in Later Life

Don Ardell and Jack Welber

Praise for *Not Dead Yet*

Not Dead Yet, written by two of USA Triathlon's most decorated senior athletes, is a testament to the benefits of staying active and open to new experiences later in life. It gives us a perspective we all need—that life at any age should be fully enjoyed—and that later life is no exception.

Don Ardell and Jack Welber truly espouse the virtues that keep us mentally young and physically capable of doing all that we aspire to do — at any age, and on all fields of play. The ensemble of others they interview for the book are among our most talented and well-versed athletes in the world and are well qualified to speak about thriving and flourishing in later life.

TIM YOUNT

Chief Sport Development Officer of USA Triathlon (USAT)

This book will inspire you! Don and Jack share some very profound, yet simple advice and practices from their interviews with world champion triathletes who are 75+. I was inspired just by reading their bios—but there is so much more to this book about how we can flourish and enjoy life to the fullest as we age. This book is a gift to those who want to age well.

DEBORAH CONNORS

Author, *A Better Place To Work: Daily Practices That Transform Culture*

This is wonderful! Truly it is. Such wit and wisdom. It's beautiful. Love it!

BILL DUNN

Editor emeritus of Freethought Today

If you are not dead yet, then this book is for you. Filled with sage advice from a bevy of seasoned experts, *Not Dead Yet* is your guide for a longer health span and a better quality of life. Now, who doesn't want that?

COLIN MILNER

CEO/Founder, International Council on Active Aging

It's my pleasure to offer a commentary on this very insightful book! I know all the contributors. The editors have put together a brilliant collection of messages for our minds and bodies.

Not Dead Yet offers life direction and sound advice. I shared the contents with my three kids in their twenties and my 95-year-old Dad! *NDY* transcends all ages!

Aging is usually described as a decline in brain and body function. Contrary to this misaligned notion, *NDY* takes an opposite view. The book provides a recipe for those who wish to nourish, thrive and elevate their health as they age. The tips on offer are paths to physical, emotional and psychological harmony.

As a mid-60's aging athlete, I think the gift of *Not Dead Yet* is to spark hope, passion and a will to embrace life as we age. Don and Jack are gems in describing this journey.

DAVE SCOTT

Six-time Pro Ironman World Champion
First person inducted in the Ironman Hall of Fame

All the tips are helpful and sound—a few will knock your socks off.

COLLEEN DE REUCK

Four-time Olympian & former world record holder 10 mile & 20K

Not Dead Yet offers great tips for mindfulness and wellbeing from those who have experienced much of what life has to offer. The participants have overcome many challenges. They share their personal formulas for overall success and happiness. *NDY* is an easy but must read!

SIMON LESSING
Five-time Pro World Triathlon Champion

Most older people end up in age care and dementia wards, drooling, making little sense. It's the reward we mostly achieve for staying alive way too long, winning only diminished life quality. Not so the 18 participants in *NDY*. They are the true masters of their own domain. They are some of the rare people who chose to become fit, think well and die healthy.

GRANT DONOVAN
Author, *Wellness Orgasms: The Fun Way to Live Well and Die Healthy*

18 world champions share their experiences in this masterpiece of guidance for healthy lives. I found it meaningful to read their advice on one of the hardest of all challenges, namely, to treat yourself well, especially in the face of so many distractions. This book is a great read!

RAPHAEL V. LUPO
Attorney & Fan of *Not Dead Yet*

The advice for thriving and flourishing now as well as in one's later life by 18 superbly fit octogenarian athletes is a compelling guide that should be recommended by doctors, teachers, employers and, for that matter, our government. It is convincing, utterly sensible, sweeping in scope, inspirational and, perhaps best of all, fun to read.

DAVID RANDLE
Managing Director - Blue Community

Dedications

Don

To daughter and son Jeanne and Jon, to grandchildren Charlie, Cadence and Buddy Miles and to my dear wife Carol, the great loves of my life.

Jack

To the memory of my father Phillip and mother Rose for benign and loving neglect; to my oldest brother Irwin for sharing wisdom; to my son Philip for demonstrating resilience; to my daughter Audrey for courage and to my wife Emelia for being there, always, with unspoken deeds of love.

Note: While banned in Saudi Arabia, forbidden at the Trump White House and condemned by L'Osservatore Romano, this edition is non-redacted, uncensored, unblacklisted, unexpurgated and uninhibited, the better for readers like you.

Table of Contents

Foreword   Stephen Jonas, MD

Preface   Audience
                         The Nature of Thriving and Flourishing

Chapter One   Introduction: Meet the Participants
                         Four REAL Wellness Dimensions

Chapter Two   Reason Dimension: Tips for Decision-Making
                         Based Upon Facts, Evidence and Science

Chapter Three   Exuberance Dimension: Tips for Happiness
                         and Joy, Meaning and More

Chapter Four   Athleticism Dimension: Tips for Sound
                         Nutrition and Vigorous Daily Exercise

Chapter Five   Liberty Dimension: Tips for Personal
                         Freedoms That Enable You to Realize Your
                         Desires, Interests and Preferences

Chapter Six   Biographies & Epilogue

Appendix   List of the 56 Tips by Number
                         Acknowledgements
                         Recommended Readings

Foreword

If you are reading this Foreword, you are *Not Dead Yet*.
But, what does that mean? Are you hanging around, somewhat active physically and mentally, but not in any sense exceptional, out of the ordinary?

All well and good if normalcy is the goal, but maybe you'd like to know more about getting to a higher level. Perhaps instead of mitigating declines or even just maintaining your quality of life, maybe, even at your age, you could improve things considerably by raising your expectations and commitment to wellbeing.

As you age chronologically, perhaps you can regain and extend your once youthful vitality by becoming younger functionally. We all age, but not at the same rate, as this book dramatically suggests.

I've written many books on health, wellness and multi-sport racing (e.g., triathlon and duathlon). At age 82, I'm now in my 37th season in these sports, having done over 250 races. I have, as you might expect, developed my own approaches to healthy aging, nearly all of which closely align with the philosophy and tips in *Not Dead Yet*. However, there is one big difference between me and the writers of this book, many of whom I have had the privilege of knowing personally. They are all fast—all are national and world champions. I have never been accused of being fast nor would anyone with any sense flatter me with such a canard. I am not fast. I always finish at the back of the pack. I'm naturally slow in all three sports—I've never had to work at it.

I participate and I finish. And I owe my longevity in the sport to healthy aging, to the principles and concepts that bind this marvelous collection of 56 tips for thriving and flourishing.

Don, it should be noted, was the first health care professional to take the term wellness, originally developed in a little-known book by Dr. Halbert Dunn in 1961, and project the concept onto the national stage. In a fine, fun book 50 years later, Don and Jack describe REAL wellness tips in this highly readable text.

We all recognize that human bodies deteriorate and decline, naturally. What we try to do with REAL wellness choices is slow the speed and direction of inevitable frailties. Many adults, throughout all life stages including advanced seniority, have turned their lives around in positive ways, mentally and physically. *Not Dead Yet* shows that later life can be the most enjoyable stage of life.

STEVEN JONAS, M.D., M.P.H.
Author, *Triathloning for Ordinary Mortals*

Preface

Audience

Not Dead Yet is for everyone in midlife and beyond who wants to be fit and well or, as we say, thriving and flourishing. The alternative, the norm, is a frail or feeble *senior-hood*, but in most instances, it need not be. We are capable of reaching later life mentally and physically able, fully prepared to enjoy the retirement decades.

Not Dead Yet is modeled after and shaped by the experiences of 18 world triathlon champions, all over 75 years of age. Their 56 practical tips based upon their personal experiences and observations identify the mindsets and actions we believe matter most for thriving and flourishing in the later years. We're confident the principles outlined will appeal to, work for and benefit all age groups. The 56 tips will serve those older now and benefit those young still, at present and when they are young no more.

Speaking of young no more, readers should take heart. As Malachy McCourt observed, *death need not be fatal. When you stop getting older, you're dead.* (That quote makes no sense, but it made us laugh when we heard it!) We prefer something Robert Green Ingersoll said about being young no more, namely: *It is hard to live a great while without growing old, and it is hardly worthwhile to die just to stay young.*

The Nature of Thriving

To thrive, flourish and thoroughly enjoy later life means to function effectively while experiencing ample meaning, delighted to be alive and active. A goal all might consider is to live in ways that render retirement years the best of life's stages.

While sound medical advice and high-quality care are important throughout life, *Not Dead Yet* is entirely focused on staying well and becoming healthier, for as long as humanly possible. This book offers no remedies for illnesses—only strategies, insights and skills that tend to prevent and/or delay declines while promoting thriving and flourishing.

Not Dead Yet draws on the insights of successful, dynamic senior athletes who have enjoyed and continue to delight in living after successful business, medical, military and other careers. It outlines a wide range of ways that you can boost your chances to do so as well.

Being an older person in top form is an achievement. Those who manage it have overcome a lifetime of trials and challenges. Think of all the random and other events and circumstances that could have put an end to you over the course of multiple decades. Now it's time to celebrate by enjoying every day of it. Welcome to *Not Dead Yet*!

The Realities of Aging

Many perennials and near-perennials remember Bob Dylan's 1964 song *My Back Pages*, particularly the refrain, *Ah, but I was so much older then, I'm younger than that now*. The tune is sometimes played at our presentations to make the point that we all have two ages, one decided at birth – that's our chronological age and it can't be changed. Many people obsess about their chronological age—a pity, since it's fixed. But, there's another that gets too little attention—that is our REAL wellness age. This is what matters because it's highly modifiable. The 56 tips in *Not Dead Yet* all celebrate the latter. Those wonderful lines, *Ah, but I was so much older then, I'm younger than that, now*, is what *Not Dead Yet* is all about. Most of the tips, if followed, will help you become younger now than your chronological age might suggest. Focus on functional abilities, not static age.

Don and Jack would like to think that, if the great 19th century editor/writer Alice Hubbard could read *NDY*, she would proclaim, as she did about another work in her time, that it's *a book without myth, miracle, mystery or metaphysics — a commonsense work for people who prize*

12

commonsense. The Great Lady believed books that benefit most are those that inspire readers to think and act for themselves. She said, *the world can only be redeemed through action, movement and motion. Un-coerced, un-bribed and un-bought. With these qualities, humanity might move toward the light.* Admittedly, the authors get carried away at times. They also like to think Charles Darwin might have said, *Damn, NDY is better than 'On the Origin of Species by Means of Natural Selection'!*

The 56 *Not Dead Yet* tips were composed in this spirit—to guide readers to evolve with the light of reason, exuberant experiences and maximum freedom. Better younger now in ways that really count. Whether fit or fat, active or sedentary, successful or struggling, we will all face a myriad of age-related changes, some welcome, many not. The welcome changes are modest—lesser duties and expectations, more leisure and perhaps boosts in quality of life. The unwelcome changes are ultimately dramatic if gradual—poorer physical and mental health, loss of connections and a future initially dim that grows progressively worse. Sportswriter Jason Gay marveled at a long-term (13-year) contract given to a star baseball player, noting that *not a single one of us is promised so much as tomorrow,* adding *this is life. When you think about it, we're all technically on short-term deals.*

While we can't change realities, we can better the odds for effective adaptations that extend enjoyments in later life.

The 18 women and men profiled in this book share two salient characteristics: 1) the benefit of good fortune - the single most vital ingredient for successful aging; and 2) lifestyle qualities known to promote successful aging. All are currently experiencing the culminating phase of their lives and doing so in a manner worthy of note. They share positive, optimistic expectations for advanced senior-hood.

That, in any case, is the overarching goal of this publication. Scholars of human affairs believe that history is difficult to appreciate at the time it is being made. This observation seems applicable to growing older - it's not noticeable at first, and acceptance and adaptations are often too long delayed. Rectifying that situation is another goal of *Not Dead Yet.*

There are many differences between this book and the overwhelming literature on aging that crowd bookstore shelves. One is that *NDY* celebrates positive, successful aging; the participants do not dwell upon the myriad negative aspects of growing old.

Another is that many if not most of the 56 tips will inform, motivate and guide your decisions in the potential-filled years from here on out. And now it's time to meet the participants.

Chapter One

Introduction: Meet the Participants

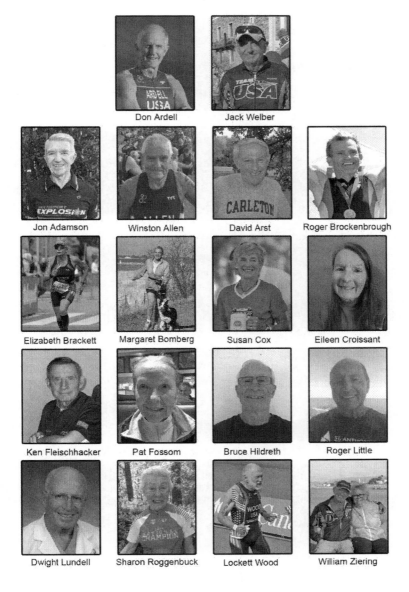

Don Ardell

Jack Welber

Jon Adamson

Winston Allen

David Arst

Roger Brockenbrough

Elizabeth Brackett

Margaret Bomberg

Susan Cox

Eileen Croissant

Ken Fleischhacker

Pat Fossom

Bruce Hildreth

Roger Little

Dwight Lundell

Sharon Roggenbuck

Lockett Wood

William Ziering

The tips and all else in the book represent nearly 1,500 years-worth of insights gained over the course of 1,000+ triathlons and a wide range of careers and otherwise varied life experiences.

This is a good deal more than anyone might expect from a single author, or two for that matter.

The 56 recommendations in *Not Dead Yet* represent the collected insights of 18 world triathlon champions, all over 75, world class athletes and accomplished men and women who worked with Don and Jack for over a year of interviews, phone calls, weekly emails and, in many cases, personal interactions at races and elsewhere.

The 18 seniors profiled herein had multiple opportunities for over a year to contribute to, read and comment on every tip and word that appears in this book. This, of course, does not mean everyone agrees with every idea expressed herein, for that certainly is not the case. Responsibility rests solely with Don and Jack, the co-authors who, though far apart geographically (Florida and Colorado, respectively), were in near-daily contact and came together, eventually, on the language herein and every decision made from inception of the idea to the publication of this book.

The participants are a varied and accomplished lot. You'll find individual biographies of the 18 in Chapter Six.

All are college graduates, most with advanced degrees. Three are medical doctors, two attorneys, two engineers, three company CEOs, two health care administrators, a pharmaceutical executive/headhunter and five coaches. All seem to have done well in their professional as well as athletic capacities.

In addition, the group includes a reporter, a musician and six veterans.

A few unusual participant factoids include the following:

- Susan Bradley-Cox and Roger L. Brockenbrough have been inducted into the USA Triathlon Hall of Fame.
- Don Ardell has two patents; Roger Little and Lockett Wood hold multiple patents.
- Five of our world triathlon champions did not take up competitive exercise until they were in their 50s or later; a few (Winston Allen, Susan and Don, were members of university athletic teams for diving, synchronized swimming/gymnastics and basketball, respectively).
- An annual triathlon in Kentucky is named in honor of one *Not Dead Yet* contributor (Susan Bradley-Cox) and

another (Bill Ziering) runs a ministry for families in financial need.

Finally, just in case you wondered, none of the participants is incarcerated, wanted by the F.B.I. or married to more than one person. They all vote, pay taxes and are kind to animals.

As co-authors, we can testify that they are all nice people, and we hope you meet one or more of them someday. But, don't put it off too long.

Use this book to accomplish much more than simply being *not dead yet*: let it be a guide to vibrant liveliness and delight in later life well beyond the mediocrity of traditional societal expectations. A high-quality lifestyle consistent with REAL wellness principles will enable mental and physical vitality for extended periods beyond the norms of aging.

The team of champion *perennials* (a term we occasionally apply for relief from such tired labels as *seniors, elders, old timers, superannuators* or, worst of all, the *pre-dead*) prefers to emphasize action--behaviors that implement forward-moving advice. *Not Dead Yet* is wholly designed to foster health-enhancing actions that add wellbeing and enjoyment beyond the absence of discomfort, limitations and suffering. The 56 tips that follow embrace the bright side of perennial life, practical ways to bring a bit of spring and summer to the fall and winter of existence.

Enjoy the words of wisdom from our champion triathletes while you ponder and implement advice that strikes a chord for enriching life. Consider and experiment with as many tips as you can, little by little and bit by bit. In doing so, you'll be making the most of opportunities associated with being more mature and wiser than ever, and having more time to do what you want, with whom and when, in ways you choose to go about it. Elder life situations are rich with under-appreciated possibilities - you can do more while complaining and suffering less.

Of course, our major goal for *Not Dead Yet* is that you, the reader, will enjoy the result - a lot! We resolved early on to keep things lively, amusing on occasions and memorable. For this reason, we included occasional quotations to upgrade ideas, most of which feature a remarkable American, Robert Green Ingersoll (1833-1899). Ingersoll was known as *Colonel Bob* during the last 35 years of the 19th century in tribute to his estimable service in the Union Army during the early years of the Civil War.

One of the co-authors, namely Don, is an Ingersoll enthusiast. Don gives presentations about Ingersoll at conferences, libraries, senior centers and other venues, in part because

Ingersoll championed three of the four REAL wellness dimensions, namely, reason, exuberance and liberty. Thus, Don selected Ingersoll excerpts on happiness, family, love, life and death to complement our recommendations and perspectives. We think readers will welcome the sampling of Ingersoll provided throughout. Ingersoll is, after all, the most famous American most people (today) have never heard of.

Let us introduce this incomparable orator by summarizing his creed, a paean to happiness, a treasured quality of successful aging:

> *While I am opposed to all orthodox creeds, I have a creed myself; and my creed is this. Happiness is the only good. The time to be happy is now. The place to be happy is here. The way to be happy is to make others so. This creed is somewhat short, but it is long enough for this life, strong enough for this world. If there is another world, when we get there, we can make another creed. But this creed certainly will do for this life.* — 1882

While we cannot directly make others happy, we can and are seeking, with this book, to provide sparkling tips and commentaries that brighten days. We seek to inspire informed action to boost the likelihood that you find happiness and good health, love and joyful living in the time remaining.

Four REAL Wellness™ Dimensions

R-E-A-L wellness is a conscious lifestyle philosophy conducive to successful aging—at any age. The acronym REAL represents Reason, Exuberance, Athleticism and Liberty. REAL wellness entails thinking critically, having fun in life, eating well, becoming and staying fit and, last but not least, insisting on enough personal freedoms to live life on your own terms, at least as much as you can get away with.

REAL wellness is a lifestyle philosophy that animates and informs positive attitudes, habits and behaviors. It does not constitute a medical intervention, product or service. It involves how one thinks and acts, not what he or she obtains from outside sources.

REAL wellness is a distinctive approach to life enrichment. It encourages promotion of wellbeing, not prevention of illness, though that which increases the likelihood of greater health automatically tends to prevent or reduce the risks of sickness. REAL wellness is not a form of alternative/holistic or integrative health practice, all of which are properly associated with forms of medical intervention. In short, REAL wellness is focused on positive wellbeing, thriving and flourishing. It does not mean ignoring life's harsh realities, troubles, setbacks, crises and all the rest, nor neglecting service to others and caring for matters larger than oneself. It does invite, to the extent possible, thinking critically, being joyful and functioning with maximum freedom. No one need feel guilty for wanting life to be fun and desiring personal freedoms that enable a better life. Perhaps a REAL wellness focus will shift the public understanding of the term wellness to life enrichment and enhancement of wellbeing—the improvement of men and women. This is what Halbert L. Dunn described in his landmark *High Level Wellness* (R.W. Beatty, LTD, 1961) and, much earlier, by Robert Green Ingersoll in his 1890 address entitled, *The Improved Man.* (C.P. Farrell in *The Complete Works of Robert Green Ingersoll,* 1902).

Besides thriving and flourishing, there are related expressions for the focus of REAL wellness that emphasize its positive nature, one worthy for its own sake, independent of medical and health benefits. These include to bloom, blossom, prosper, burgeon and radiate. More awareness of REAL wellness, as described in this book, might encourage more people, at all of life's stages, to seek nothing less than a self-directed, positive orientation for life.

And now it's our pleasure to offer the 56 tips for your consideration. As Robert Ingersoll wished his musician friend Anton Siedl in signing off in a letter, *Good luck and long life, and music enough to last you through.*

Chapter Two

Reason Dimension: Tips for Decision Making Based Upon Facts, Evidence and Science

1. CHOOSE A LIFE OF DISCIPLINED EXCELLENCE

Discipline is essential if you wish to be free, live well, enjoy life and age successfully.

There are variables too numerous to list that affect success in this life, and none is more consequential than the one over which we have no control, namely, random fortune. The place and time of our birth is one example, not being on the wrong end of a lightning strike is another - there are billions of chance encounters that, for better or worse, affect how long we live, the roads we take, the jobs and professions we adopt, who we marry and so on. These are consequential occurrences that shape our fate and all are random; there is nothing logical, predictable or manageable about any of them. Crudely put, we are vastly affected by dumb luck.

Fortunately, there is much more over which we do have influence, and these are the factors that should concern us and be attended to if we wish to do well and make the most of our relatively short existence on this good Earth.

At the top of any list should be discipline, control of thoughts and actions. It is discipline that keeps us on track, enables us to manage impulses and feelings and sustains movement toward goals. Consistent success over time requires self-discipline. In a speech entitled *Improved Man*, Robert Green Ingersoll described nine major qualities, virtues, values, commitments and not common—enough common decencies that represent an improved version of men and women, hopefully at some time in the not-too-distant future. Each quality had multiple sub-qualities. Consider the ninth such quality, which in multiple ways touches on self-discipline as a key feature of being free, living well, enjoying life and yes, aging successfully:

> *The Improved Man will be self-poised, independent, candid and free. He will be a scientist. He will observe, investigate, experiment and demonstrate. He will use his sense and his senses. He will keep his mind open as the day to the hints and suggestions of nature. He will always be a student, a learner and a listener—a believer in intellectual hospitality. In the world of his brain there will be continuous summer, perpetual seedtime and harvest. Facts will be the foundation of his faith. In one hand he will carry the torch of truth, and with the other raise the fallen.*

Recently, the point was also made by Kenyan marathoner Eliud Kipchoge, age 33, who said the following about this essential ingredient of success:

> *Only the disciplined ones in life are free. If you are undisciplined, you are a slave to your moods and your passions. It's not about the legs; it's about the heart and the mind.*

He added what many believe to be a Chinese parable:

> *The best time to plant a tree was 25 years ago. The second-best time to plant a tree is today.*

Kipchoge's own discipline in life enabled him to accomplish an extraordinary feat, one that was hard for even the experts to believe. What he did rocketed him to fame on the morning of September 16, 2018, in Berlin: He shattered the world record for the marathon by running slightly over 26 consecutive miles at a pace of four minutes, 38 seconds per mile, winning the fabled event in 2:01:39. Evidently, Mr. Kipchoge is disciplined and free from his moods and passions, master of his heart and mind and well aware of the value of being self-poised. His mention of the best times to plant a tree represents an apt metaphor for aging successfully. The quote echoes Ingersoll's words from 1890: *In the world of his brain,* there will be *continuous summer, perpetual seedtime and harvest*—in abundance.

2. WELLBEING REQUIRES A HIGHLY FIT BRAIN

Load up on brain attitudinal and activity workouts, for mental acumen is the foundation for thriving and flourishing in later life.

Your perspectives, beliefs, values and other elements of personality represent who you are, how you behave and how you're perceived. All brains are initially filled with impressions from the perspectives, beliefs, values and other elements of the personalities of family and others. An adult brain that is truly fit almost certainly requires personal modifications, over time. The fine-tuning or major overhauls, depending on your early circumstances, must be based upon your own observations, investigations, experiments and demonstrations. A highly fit brain is one that you must ultimately shape for yourself. At least as much as the physical fitness that you achieve and maintain daily, the fitness of your brain will determine the extent to which you live well and enjoy the years ahead.

Varied mind games provide mental challenges that nourish the brain, the central processing unit for who you are. They can boost your problem solving, communication and social skills. Staying sharp provides multiple benefits. Skill building takes place with games such as bridge and chess, two favorites that tend to keep your wits and mental states in top working order.

As important as vigorous physical training is for Jack Welber (he works out six to seven days a week and would surely train on additional days if more were available), he recognizes that a highly fit brain also takes work. He knows the benefits are at least as dramatic as the physical returns.

Ten years of playing bridge, writing papers and listening to podcasts have led Jack to believe that his brain is still in fine working order, and most of us who know him agree. Among his favorite podcasts are Sam Harris' *Making Sense* and Dan Carlin's *Hardcore History*. He realizes it's not enough to learn the fundamentals of bridge, chess, writing and so on; mental discipline exerted in order to get better at them is invaluable. For one thing, others enjoy the game more if all play well; for another, you have more fun if your game is well regarded. Mental workouts of all kinds require time and energy to derive the most from them.

Roger Brockenbrough also noted the value of brain workouts. He mentioned staying sharp with crossword puzzles— stretching to find that special word benefits mental flexibility and agility. Roger extols the merits of deep thinking, regularly going beyond the routine application of knowledge. The stimulating effects of engaging with colleagues in search of a solution to a technical problem is as beneficial as physical exercise.

Sports involve multiple challenges requiring a clear head. An example well known to the champion participants in this book is the sport of triathlon. In this multiple-activity endeavor, the athlete must juggle disparate requirements. These include remembering to bring a variety of equipment to the race site, getting in and out of the playing field (i.e., the transition areas) as expeditiously as possible and knowing when to hold and when to fold them. By that we mean when to make strategic moves to advance under dramatically different circumstances.

Triathlons commence with a scrum when the starter's signal sends competitors off on the initial swim leg of the race. Space gets tight as the first turn-buoy nears, as swimmers seek to be as close as possible to the buoy. The entire swim requires moving forward in deep, sometimes troubled waters, frequently jostling for position. With the swim ordeal complete, a run to transition and quick change into biker mode follows. Again, the start is tricky and hazardous, as many frantic cyclists hurriedly attempt to mount their steeds and set off without hitting others attempting to do likewise.

The bike portion of a triathlon offers some degree of serenity, especially when the course is relatively flat or rolling and hairpin turns, suicidal descents and/or reckless competitors are not present. Next comes the run. This is the safest but most exhausting of the three legs, especially if you are seeking podium glory or for other reasons are determined to leave your last bit of oxygen on the course at the finish line. By the time you depart transition for the final run segment, your energy resources are in serious decline, diminishing with each stride. Mental acuity is essential: The serious competitor wants to reach the finish line nearly exhausted. Hold back too much and you could lose a place or two; spend too much before you reach the Promised Land (i.e., the finish line) and you might drop dead, or at least abandon ship (i.e., quit the race). In other words, while bodily fitness matters, so too does mental acuity.

However, the satisfaction in doing all of this safely and well over the course of one to several hours is considerable, self-confidence is strengthened and you feel that all's right with the world.

Everything's relative, and some endeavors make triathlon competitions seem like the proverbial walk in the park.

Would you like an example? Here's one to think about - climbing the near-vertical 3,000-foot El Capitan wall in

Yosemite National Park - without a harness or other safety equipment. Choosing not to consider such a thing does not, however, inhibit us to a point where we can't be dazzled by and appreciative of the skills and fortitude of someone like American climber Alex Honnold who, in 2017, ascended this exact El Capitan wall - without ropes or a parachute! National Geographic magazine described Mr. Honnold's free solo climb on June 3 as perhaps the greatest feat of pure rock climbing in the history of the sport.

We old guys and gals think it's more like the greatest feat of anything, ever, in the whole wide world. But, who knows? Maybe we're just easily impressed!

Lest you think that brain nourishment requires heroic feats or just plain strenuous physical exertions, know that using your mind qualifies, too. Writing, for example, is another quite different but still nutrient-rich way to nourish the brain. It is valuable for self-understanding and for creating a record for others to appreciate who you are - and later, who you were. Otherwise, special times, events and experiences known only to and felt only by you might go unrecorded, forevermore.

3. IF YOU ARE AGING WELL, SHARE YOUR TIPS

No need to write a book about it, like some people, but spread the wealth.

You might want to start by expressing your views, insights and/or theories on what's involved in dealing with physical changes that accompany getting older. Tell friends what you have deduced from your long experience at aging and consider what they have to offer on such matters. Offer a few tips for successful aging - you're welcome to embellish any of ours, if so inclined.

Besides sharing your knowledge, continue developing your skills for evidence-based thinking. Employ the reasoning capacity you gained over a lifetime to help others think rationally in order that they, too, can repulse the flim-flam artists, vulgarians and deplorables political, religious, economic and otherwise. Pass along your wisdom in order to help others make decisions not based upon dysfunctional traditions, gut instincts, group pressures, excessive testosterone levels or plain immaturity. Master and share a few common-sense, reason-based techniques with others.

Continue to build and stockpile decision skills with continuing education - and remain current on events, controversies and other matters that seem likely to affect your quality of life and your ability to work with others. Jon Adamson coaches athletes, all of whom are younger than himself. Here's his advice consistent with the tip at hand:

Given all the technological advances, the apps and extensive software in use by the young, I have to maintain a strong command of these developments to be effective as a coach. This helps motivate me to study and learn continuously.

If you have the heart for it, make a scene - show up at town council meetings, write or call your politicians, submit letters-to-the-editor, vote and engage in discussions about public policies, the arts and the dynamics of contemporary life. Don't be shy about telling stories, creatively embellished, if necessary, to hold audience attention. If you are a senior, all the better, for many of the young are innocent of the nature of life half a dozen or more decades ago. Who knows? Maybe you will dazzle these young'uns with tall tales and *based on a true story* about the dramas of your heyday.

4. DANGER - HAZMAT ALERT REGARDING THE USE AND DISPOSITION OF PILLS

Prescriptions can be perilous - treat pills and all medications as you would sticks of dynamite. Pat Fossum suggests an alternative *potion* - laughter, which is rumored to be the best medicine, free and readily available, especially if you and your friends are *afflicted* with a hearty sense of humor.

On a less humorous note, we should add more to this tip, such as keep meds away from children, always let doctors know what products you are taking and dispose of drugs as you would radioactive waste - safely where others won't be tempted to recycle them. Also, don't watch drug commercials - these deceptive and usually jejune fake dramas would not be allowed on TV or other media if one of us were the U.S. Surgeon General - or benevolent ruler of the universe. (Yes, we know the U.S. Surgeon General does not have such power - we're just being a little dramatic to get our point across.)

Until the mid-80s, pharmaceutical companies were not permitted to pitch drugs directly to consumers, as they do today. Drug ads were designed for doctors through private channels, not for lay customers via mass media. Advertising of medications was originally created by technically minded, medically focused ad agencies - and targeted only to small, mostly doctor audiences. Now ads are designed for consumers who have no clue as to how to assess the value of such products or the risks of same; the purpose of such ads is only to motivate consumers to pressure doctors to prescribe drug products they've seen on TV. Those (paid actors) depicted in the ad dramas always seem to get better after taking the product at hand, and also seem happier and more energetic than ever before - and thus ever so willing to praise the product without reservation.

More than anything else, drug ads should be seen as public service messages demonstrating the need for critical thinking skills. As you well know, that's probably the last thing pharmaceutical companies would want.

Any idea how much was spent by drug makers on direct-to-consumer advertising last year? The total was $6.4 billion. Direct to consumer (DTC) advertising of pharmaceutical products increased dramatically in 1997 due to a change in the Food and Drug Administration's (FDA) regulatory policy. It is the third-largest class of televised product advertising in the US. (Source: Nielsen, 2014 and NIH Library of Medicine, 2015.)

Resistance is not futile. To age successfully, be wary, skeptical and on guard about drugs! A medication here and there can be marvelously beneficial, but only under certain conditions. Never assume meds will offer more good than harm and always do due diligence before taking such substances. To be a bit specific (a couple of our champions are physicians), some meds adversely affect the brain in the near-term while risking Alzheimer's over a longer haul. Other drugs have equally dramatic risk factors - think of the current crisis with synthetic opioids, such as fentanyl and pain relievers (e.g., oxycodone, hydrocodone, codeine and morphine).

Of course, some drugs are effective, if suitably prescribed after an accurate diagnosis of need. One of us (Don) takes an anticoagulant twice daily that is designed to prevent blood clots from forming due to his irregular heartbeat condition known as atrial fibrillation. Don takes this medication because his medical advisers and own research suggest it's the best way, in his case, to lower the risk of stroke, not because of the brain-dead ads that promote even the worthwhile medication he relies upon.

Bottom line with meds - caution is always prudent. Limit prescription and other medication usage to the extent possible - and discontinue those not deemed essential by qualified medical authorities as soon as possible.

5. BE OPTIMISTIC - PERHAPS ALL IS FOR THE BEST, BUT VERIFY

Optimism is a splendid quality; it is much to be preferred over its opposite, pessimism.

More often than not, even being overly optimistic is better than being pessimistic, but within reason. It's the how, when, why and for what optimism is felt that determines if it is a positive or negative state.

As a general rule, however, it is best to be more of an optimist like Dr. Pangloss than a pessimistic, horribilizing *megalochrondriac.*

Perhaps you're not familiar with the latter neologism, or with Voltaire's memorable character in the novel *Candide*. Dr. Pangloss is a philosopher and the main character's mentor. Pangloss is an over-the-top optimist who spoke the novel's most famous line, *All is for the best in this, the best of all possible worlds.*

Megalochondria is a new word, and it is more or less the medical opposite of an optimistic outlook. It applies to a condition wherein a person believes that his symptom or illness is far worse than it actually is. While we don't want anyone to go all Pangloss - as in looking on the bright side of everything, it's important to avoid the other extreme as well. This is so not just regarding medical matters but in other ways. For instance, when you're feeling a bit under the proverbial weather, don't go on about it such that your spouse, relatives or friends suspect you're becoming a bit like Chicken Little. Resist horribilizing - be more like Dr. Pangloss, but not too much more. That could be wearisome, too. Strike a near-balance between optimism and pessimism but tip the scale in favor of optimism. (By the way, credit for the neologism *megalochrondriac* that combines magalomania and hypochondria goes to Shannon O'Hara of Chicago, Illinois, as seen in A.Word.A.Day's *AWADmail,* Issue 829, May 20, 2018.)

6. APPRECIATE BEING ALIVE NOW, DURING THE 21ST CENTURY

Well done in timing your existence to coincide with the most advantageous of times, when the chances for successful aging are greater than ever before.

We humans of the Homo sapiens species have been around (at least in East Africa) for about 150,000 years, according to credible sources, such as Yuval Noah Harari (see *Sapiens: A Brief History of Humankind*, Harper, 2015, p. 14). For at least the past 70,000 years, we have had access to knowing more, having more and fearing less than at any time since we came to be. As of this writing, there are no world wars, global epidemics affecting most of the planet or other widespread perturbations such as have plagued mankind for the past twenty centuries and surely long before that. In his 2018 best seller, *Enlightenment Now: The Case for Reason, Science, Humanism and Progress,* Steven Pinker shows that poverty, crime, and drug abuse are declining in this country, and that our educational system, despite many serious problems, is nonetheless one of the best anywhere. Throughout the world, health status has improved, infant and maternal mortality are lower than ever, children are better fed, treated and educated. Workers have more income, get hurt less than before and have more money and, significantly for present purposes, retire earlier.

However, a case could also be made for gloom and doom, given the reality of climate change and the large-scale reluctance by one political party in the U.S. to accept the science that deeply concerns nearly every scientist in the world. Oh well, we're trying to look on the bright side here.

Living with good prospects of someday becoming a senior is a relatively new phenomenon. Make the most of your good fortune in being alive now rather than during an epoch when life really was solitary, poor, nasty, brutish - and quite short. Reliable skeletal evidence suggests the average lifespan during Greek and Roman times centuries ago was approximately 20 to 35 years. This, of course, was due not so much to the poor lifestyle patterns (the key factor that accounts for the high rates of chronic disease in our time), but rather to high infant mortality. Those who survived childbirth and early life hazards did not die of heart disease, cancer, chronic lower respiratory disease, stroke, Alzheimer's or diabetes. The causes of death were infectious diseases, from fighting and from infected wounds, accidents and unhygienic living conditions. Also consequential was having little to no effective medical care.

Lockett Wood, while recognizing that tremendous work is still required, pointed out that the U.S. is still the environmentally cleanest country in the world, something we should all appreciate. He added the following:

Medical progress in all areas is remarkable. Only a few decades ago, a cancer diagnosis was a death sentence. Many cancers are now treatable, and a complete cure is a possibility. Just years ago, there was no treatment for ischemic stroke. Today, with timely intervention, complete recovery is a realistic hope. In recent times, heart disease treatments have extended the life of millions. A close friend flatlined while riding his bicycle to work. Fortunately, there were two intensive care nurses in the car behind when he went down who provided CPR until he was transported. Two heart surgeries later he emerged healthy with no brain damage. He's currently incredibly fit and dedicated to his aerobic workouts. Only a very few years ago survival would have been impossible.

Bottom line - recognize and make the most of the wonder of your presence now as well as here, on Earth of all places, during the 21st century.

7. SEEK COMPANIONS WHO ARE RATIONAL

Reason is the mistress and queen of all things. (Marcus Tullius Cicero, Roman statesman)

Be highly selective - avoid those obsessed with conspiracy theories. No doubt you're familiar with a few, such as that an elite cohort of reptiles rule the earth, Justin Bieber among them, or that the recent ice bucket challenge was a Satanic ritual, or that Queen Elizabeth is a cannibal or that the Earth is flat and so on. (Source: Zoë Bernard, *The Craziest Conspiracy Theories on the Internet,* Business Insider, Nov. 19, 2017.)

One reason for such thinking is that many people derive pleasure and profit from making susceptible, otherwise normal but vulnerable folks a little crazy. As Eric Idle put the matter in the first stanza of the song *Always Look on the Bright Side of Life* in the immortal final scene of Monty Python's *Life of Brian*:

> *Some things in life are bad, they can really make you mad, other things just make you swear and curse.*

Fortunately, far more people are cheerful, positive and fun than the sort who make you swear and curse, or otherwise prove to be rather a pain in the derrière. Seek out the former and eschew the latter. There is not enough time left to squander any of it with those who are vexatious, tiresome, boring or mean. And let's face it - there are plenty of older people who, often for pretty good reasons, have slid into a bitter and surly fix. If that's you, liberate yourself from grumptitude; resolve to be a charmer, like the late Mr. Rogers and Liberace, or somebody like that who oozes nice. Life is too short to waste an hour, or even a minute, on bitterness or regret.

A sure-fire way to shift to charming is to associate with positive, interesting people. With no special effort, their allure and magnetism will provoke positivity in all around them, yourself included. Henceforth, your days will seem much better. Associating with vexatious people, on the other hand, will accelerate your aging and make you constipated and difficult to be around.

Kenneth Fleischhacker, one of our world champion participants, urges readers to embrace the common decencies, particularly science, reason, love, kindness and hope as proven consolations of the world. He lamented the fact that some parts of our media and approximately 40% of our voting population seem indifferent, if not hostile, to these values. Specifically, Ken wonders,

> *Why do so many in this country reject a common-sense belief system? Within my small group of friends, all relate to and embrace the common decency values noted above.*

Ken also has a few ideas that support the usefulness of this tip:

> *During my travels, particularly around multi-sport events in this country and abroad, I experience these values, which add so much satisfaction in interactions with strangers, some who become new friends. Let's teach our children and train*

ourselves to question and explore possibilities. Ask important questions that invite constructive and revealing answers that help us to explore critical thinking and promote lifelong learning. Don't passively accept information or embrace slogans or target outsiders as the cause of all tribulations in society.

8. CURB YOUR ENTHUSIASM FOR MEDICAL MIRACLES

Resist the medicalization of your senior years.

Excessive prescriptions, over-testing, unnecessary and dangerous treatments are the norm for seniors, whether athletic or not. The pressure to medicate and over-rely upon doctors comes not only from advertising, as described in a previous tip, but also from physicians and other medical personnel, family, friends and associates. It's not a plot, just a culture out of sync with and in denial about the limits of medicine and the realities of human decline in the final years. There is no cure, no fix or treatment for the wear and tear and ultimate obsolescence of body parts. However, with discipline, awareness and commitment to REAL wellness habits, you should be able to compress senescence and expand vitality beyond the norms and expectations of society.

Bruce Hildreth, a physician who practiced emergency medicine for 30 years, suggests being wary of medical miracles. Here's why, in his words:

> *I know there are few absolutes but it's important to know how to put the odds in most situations in your favor. Anecdotes are available about the success or failure of most any position. But good decisions about important things require careful investigation and consideration of the available information. And lots of information is now available about matters medical, from meds to operations and much more. Documentation of facts is more difficult than taking opinions as such, and there are always conflicting views. The phrase 'If it sounds too good to be true…' applies here. Be a skeptic. Get second and maybe third opinions. Ask lots of questions. Read studies published in reliable journals. Alternative medicine has a place and has helped thousands. But almost, as a general rule, I would suggest that you give traditional medicine a first shot at solving any problem. Traditional medicine has its own policing problems, but alternative medicine has woefully few safeguards.*

9. WHENEVER LIFE GETS YOU DOWN, THINK BIG

Think about the bigger picture—don't dwell on the small stuff. Set your sights on thriving, not surviving. You've overcome so much over the years. Your brain is filled with good memories—and no doubt memories not so appealing—focus on the present. Consider momentary step-backs as useful learning experiences not to be repeated or mourned.

This strategy can be effective under trying circumstances, such as described in Monty Python's *the Galaxy Song*:

> *Whenever things get you down ... and things seem hard or tough, and people are stupid, obnoxious or daft and you feel that you've had quite enough…*

That's when it's time to think about the bigger picture.

You know - how the planet, galaxy and universe are evolving, revolving, orbiting, moving, going around and expanding at speeds over distances that seem hard to imagine. Doing so will help you lighten up - your birth was amazing and unlikely in the first place, so make the best of being along for the ride around our sun at 19 miles a second, so it's reckoned. You don't have to agree with someone to have a dialogue, or to show that you appreciate him or her and are tolerant of views at odds with your own.

Of course, there are exceptions, but we're going to resist going off on a tangent about our presidential situation.

10. MUTE THE ADS

Be skeptical of all advertising, not just drug advertising, as already emphasized.

Take no ads at face value. None are objective; few are honest or reliable. More than not, they are misleading and/or deceptive.

The multibillion-dollar medical treatment industry appeals to emotion, not reason. In seeking customers, hyperbole is served without asterisks, except in fine print or fast-paced disclaimers. An MD Anderson Cancer Center ad proclaims, *come to us and you will beat cancer.* (Steve Salerno, In *War on Cancer, Truth Becomes a Casualty*, WSJ, April 21, 2018, p. A13.) Such a promise is fraudulent—there is no sure cure for cancer; no doctor or medical institution can fulfill a promise to the contrary.

Such ads are, however, part of a high-stakes competition for billings projected to reach $207 billion by 2020. A study published in the *Annals of Internal Medicine* in 2014 noted that cancer advertising direct to potential customers, often with celebrity pitchmen, relies on emotional appeals. Such ads evoke hope or fear while promoting expensive treatments, not screenings. The risks of treatments are noted in less than 2% of ads. The cancer industry, in short, is widely accused of exploiting false hope. Be aware that there is no condition that medical personnel, if encouraged to find a cure at all costs, can't introduce for one additional *Hail Mary* fix, however improbable. Even the most seemingly hopeless situation can usually be viewed as possibly responsive to some untested remedy, an experimental treatment, an alternative, complementary or unconventional approach, that someone, somewhere has developed with promising results.

Be skeptical. Don't be easily fooled or lured to irrational choices inspired more by false hope than reason or evidence.

11. HIGH-RISK, LOW-RETURN INITIATIVES—FORGET ABOUT THEM

Reason skills will, among other payoffs, protect you from making awful decisions. Effective decision-making knowledge put to practice will facilitate wise choices, to state the same point in a positive way.

Before doing something that seems hazardous, identify a few criteria to use for your own personal risk-taking cost/benefit assessments. Chances are you have not thought much about such criteria, so start with this single criterion: The benefits of an activity should entail substantial pleasures lasting longer than the thrill of an amusement ride. We're all in favor of adventures, trying new things, world travel and actions that topple stereotypes about aging. Resist taking on something new and unfamiliar if a judgment error or unforeseen contingency could bring ruin. You certainly don't want to take risks to impress others, like grandchildren, or to imitate youthful vitality.

What kinds of risks might we have in mind? It doesn't matter - what matters are the things you're tempted to do that involve significant dangers. But, for illustrative purposes, we'll mention a few that, despite some appeal or advantage, have ghastly consequences if things go badly:

- Flying on third-world airlines.
- Visiting countries under authoritarian rule (e.g., the Philippines, Russia, Iran, Venezuela, Zimbabwe, Saudi Arabia—there are almost a hundred others).
- Ordering Sannakji in Korean restaurants (Sannakji is a serving of live baby octopus that fights back when you swallow it by suctioning itself to your throat), or eating wild mushrooms or African bullfrogs.
- Bungee-jumping, skydiving, heli-skiing (backcountry style via helicopter drop-offs), motorcycle racing or just being on a motorcycle and a lot of events featured in the Winter Olympics, though we have nothing against curling.

Pondering these examples of jejune things people do reminds us of something physicist and cosmologist George Gamow said, namely, that *it took less than an hour to make the atoms, a few hundred million years to make the stars and planets but five billion years to make man!*

But, never mind—the *NDY* folks suggest it's better to look ahead to the glorious next stage of human evolution.

12. SURGERIES: TO BE OR NOT TO BE (OPERATED ON)

Rely on your critical-thinking skills to weigh the pros and cons of any surgery more invasive than having a tooth filled - and always seek independent advice when doctors recommend an operation.

Not much is known about the number of invasive interventions an average American endures in a lifetime, but you can be sure the figures increase considerably with age. Taking account of the significant risks of all surgeries, due diligence is highly recommended. The American College of Surgeons (Massachusetts Chapter) conducted a study in 2002 to assess the number of surgical procedures a typical American undergoes in a lifetime. The resulting report, written by Peter Lee, Scott Regenbogen and Atul A. Gawande at Caritas St. Elizabeth's Medical Center in Boston, put the number at 9.2 surgical procedures. The most common are coronary angioplasty, wound debridement and groin hernia repair for men; cesarean section, cholecystectomy and lens and cataract surgery for women.

Not surprising, the per capita rate increases considerably after age 75, though data for that statistic were not collected. There are 18 champions profiled in *Not Dead Yet*. Their legacies, like yours, include many modest if unremarked acts of personal heroism. Occasionally, these actions become elements of one's legacy. We see this with seniors when decisions involve risks taken to recapture elements of life still within range, despite the weight of many years.

Pat Fossum reported her good fortune in finding a physical therapist early in her years of triathlon training. With expert guidance, she could pinpoint the causes of concerns and employ non-invasive solutions. These precautions and treatments usually strengthened Pat's weaker muscles and the most nagging problems usually disappeared.

Sometimes such actions do not work out as hoped. We can appreciate the fortitude shown in mounting such attempts. Sometimes bold initiatives are taken to live life on one's own terms, to regain a measure of functional youth, an attempt, one more time, to grasp a treasured level of vitality, despite long odds.

An example of this phenomenon was offered by one of our senior champions, 89-year-old physician Bill Ziering. Bill decided to undergo risky back surgery a year ago in hopes of finding relief from conditions that interfered with normal functioning and eliminated any chance to return to a competitive level in the sport he loved and in which he excelled— triathlon. Just one year earlier than facing back surgery, Bill won his division in the Olympic distance event in Rotterdam. Tempted to regain this level of vitality, Bill elected to go for a fix.

This is how Bill reported on the initial outcome in an update to our small society of *Not Dead Yet* champions:

> *Man down! The roof caved in. Took a shot with surgery - spinal stenosis. Bad choice. Wound up in ICU, then to neurosurgical ward. Something went awry - clots in lungs and legs. Followed by a bit of pneumonia. Now homing at a skilled nursing center. But all that was yesterday. Today brings a new beginning since there's nothing left to befall me. The demons have given up.*

Was this choice a legacy-worthy decision? That's a matter of opinion. A distinguished physician who initially specialized in pediatrics and later allergy and respiratory medicine, Dr. Bill knew well the risks, which were judged acceptable. He weighed the hazards and went ahead - with eyes wide open and faith that a good outcome was a possibility. The bottom line for Bill was the desire to do what had to be done to have any hope of recapturing the capacity to experience something deeply valued. Surgery seemed within the range of possibilities, despite the weight of years.

Now Bill will move on, continuing to do the best that can be done, under new circumstances.

Oh, by the way, he registered and is training for the coming world championship in Lausanne, Switzerland. Bravo, Dr. Bill.

13. SURGERY IS A GAMBLE

Odds should be high that surgery will improve your quality of life, not just extend your survival at the margins.

Dr. Ziering now identifies as *a slow-learning triathlete* based upon the above account of his experience with back surgery. He advises all athletes to keep two health files, one with medical history, medications and so on, and another with medical articles of interest.

His advice begins with the idea that we should rely only on board-certified physicians. Be sure that surgery is the last option. A chronic debilitating injury deserves an initial trial with a physiatrist (i.e., a specialist in physical medicine and rehabilitation). Daily core training at home over a period of months is another prerequisite.

Dr. Bill's recent spinal stenosis surgery, though well done, crippled him for weeks, and the prognosis is for months of lesser pain while he undergoes relearning how to walk and preparing for the next big triathlon!

Other elements of his advice to all can be summarized:

> *When biking, be entirely focused. You pay dearly for carelessness. Never push yourself to stay up with leaders and don't beat yourself up for a subpar performance. Maintain a comfortable pace. Fine if winning is your goal (after all, someone has to do it), but you might overlook the joy of the endeavor if such an aspiration becomes compulsive or frustrating. On the other hand, if joy is is your goal, you're more likely to remain in the sport forevermore, or until the end, whichever comes first.*

Join a club with like-minded athletes. Couple this tip with sound nutrition, stress management and close friendships and you will have a pathway to healthful longevity and enhanced pleasures.

Chapter Three

Exuberance Dimension: Tips That Focus on Happiness and Joy, Meanings, Purposes and More

14. GO OUT OF YOUR WAY FOR HUMOR, FUN, JOY AND HAPPINESS

Humor and its cousins—fun, joy and happiness—bring amusement, laughter, pleasure and more—all nutrients for the secular soul.

Humor is often unexpected. From our earliest days, having fun has had appeal. It's purposeful and, no surprise, is no less important and nourishing to life quality in the latter years as ever before. Fun is often unexpected and takes many forms.

Look for humor opportunities in whatever you're doing, though solemn religious devotions may be among the few occasions when others might not be enthusiastic if you're having too much fun. Nevertheless, not having enough fun could be an overlooked health hazard - serial solemnity is associated with being cranky, moody, grumpy, crabby, crotchety, testy, prickly, irascible, cantankerous, surly, peevish or simply not exactly being the life of any party.

Social scientists can't seem to say enough in favor of the health benefits of laughter as good medicine and a common feature of wellbeing. Studies of long-lived people highlight ample laughter as a characteristic of successful aging. It is beneficial even if the source of merriment is not understandably amusing. Someone who laughs incessantly, however, including at times when nothing seems funny to anyone else, is unnerving. However, if nobody's listening, go ahead and yuck it up at every opportunity. It will do no harm and, if the scientists and best-selling humor book authors are not having us on, might do some good. Around others, it's best if at least a few get the joke.

Happiness is closely related to, but different from, laughter. The latter is a sensation; happiness is a feeling, somewhat longer lasting than a hearty chuckle. Aristotle posited two forms of happiness: hedonia, based on pleasure, and eudaimonia, based on virtue and clean living. Likewise, there are two distinct kind of laughter—good natured and victimless (basically eudaimonia) and all the rest, as favored by the varieties of humor in stand-up comedy (basically hedonic). Both kinds are heartily recommended.

15. BE ADVENTURESOME

As often as you can and if it's still fun, do things you never did before. Don't worry - you'll never exhaust the possibilities.

Becoming set in your ways, uninterested in unfamiliar places, people, foods and much of anything else often leads to hesitation in so much as leaving one's house, boredom, apathy and a downhill slope. Not good - even small adventures can be life-quality saving.

This kind of slippage in life happens slowly, but it's inevitable if met with little or no resistance. When you no longer have a full head of drop-dead gorgeous hair and your back hurts and you feel tired and grumpy and you just want to be left alone to watch reruns of *I Love Lucy* or *Gunsmoke*, give a little adventure a try. Crash a party and become the life of it, or better yet, get yourself invited to a few. Accept opportunities to go places, even if the destinations are not of interest, initially, such as museums, concerts, plays, dances, bingo parties. Any function might be worth a try, since it will get you out, which will lead to mingling with others and enjoying company that might prove entertaining. Favor celebratory occasions, like graduations, award ceremonies, birthdays, weddings and conferences. Funerals are ok, now and then, but don't attend too many. Otherwise, you might find yourself obsessing about death or quoting Woody Allen: *It's not that I'm afraid to die. I just don't want to be there when it happens.*

One of our champions, Roger Brockenbrough, a structural steel engineer by profession, reported that his biggest adventure was taking an early retirement. An opportunity arose at age 57 when the steel industry was downsizing. This occurred at a time when he was fully immersed in the world of triathlon and thought how much more fun it would be if he had more personal time. Breaking ties with a 9 to 5 routine was a huge adventure for an otherwise conservative guy. But, with encouragement from family, it all worked out.

Susan Bradley-Cox wasted no time finding new adventures after stepping back from competing at the highest level in triathlon when inevitable fragilities of the body overcame the desires of her mind. She was aware of several alternatives to exercising outside the needs to prepare for competitions, including familiar outlets like swimming and biking. Hiking with friends proved to be a delightful new routine for Susan's ample energies. She also resuscitated her dormant golf game. These and other initiatives proved to be fulfilling opportunities for mixing with old friends while meeting new ones.

Whatever your circumstances, don't wait too long or let comfortable circumstances or a lack of blinding, world-class talent or other factors hold you back. Rumor has it that there are at least 10 life-enriching qualities that require no talent whatsoever, namely, being active and coachable, having an active work ethic, conscious body language and a positive attitude, effort, energy and passion doing extra and staying prepared.

16. BE BOLD, SPONTANEOUS AND GREGARIOUS

Something about aging leads many, if not most, to become overly cautious, resistant to change and noticeably withdrawn.

Sure, there are reasons for this. For example, falls are a hazard, we don't have the agility of earlier times and we get fewer invitations from the wild and crazy guys and gals who used to encourage us to go a bit beyond our comfort zones. This, not surprisingly, is because our older friends are more cautious and withdrawn themselves!

Well, turn the tables. You be the one who comes up with ideas for little outings of derring-do, edgier than you've become accustomed to of late. The rewards, if you manage such adventures intact and without terminal embarrassment, could be loads of good fun.

You never know when something great might happen by virtue of a bold move and, if you could look back on such a time, you'll be so grateful you took the risk. Consider a tale told by Lockett Wood:

> *Thirteen years after I was widowed, I was sitting at JFK Airport waiting for a flight to Denver. A beautiful woman seated across the room was waiting for the same flight. She opened a package of candy but spilled it all. I had just purchased a package of the same candy, so I walked over, laid my candy on her book and went back to my seat. After everyone was loaded, I convinced the gatekeeper to have me seated next to her on the flight. A year later we were married while running the Bolder Boulder, the famous local 10K. That was 27 years ago. It's sometimes possible to restart your life at almost any age.*

Lockett's case is not the norm. Too often, invisible dimmer switches, or what might be governors of a kind, emerge in later life on spontaneity. These cautions unnecessarily limit former interests, inhibiting gregariousness. This can be another downside of aging if not recognized and resisted.

Fortunately, such controls on exuberance, with a little conscious effort, can be overridden. The next time you are asked to do or join in on something that sounds a bit anxiety-inducing, consider accepting. It may represent an opportunity to live lively in the moment, to regain for a spell that old gregariousness or sense of daring. Don't give a thought to concern that you might suffer a little momentary embarrassment or provoke a bit of humor at your expense. In the quest for some spontaneity and delight, a little risk-taking will do scarce harm. It's not as if the consequences might be truly disastrous for all mankind, as Neil deGrasse Tyson once playfully described:

> *I don't want to be the embarrassment of the galaxy to have had the power to deflect an asteroid, and then not and end up going extinct. We'd be the laughingstock of the aliens of the cosmos if that were the case.*

There is something quite specific you could do that would almost surely render you spontaneous and bold—take an improv class—Don did and loved it. Doing so will provide you with valuable skills, boost your self-confidence and, best of all, prove to be an absolute hoot (i.e., rollicking good fun).

Improv is a fun way to tap into your creative energy while learning simple techniques useful for managing real-life stresses and challenging situations. In an improv class, you'll learn to invent something useful out of an improbable, initially irrelevant existing thing or circumstance. You will be an actor/actress able to create a story, similar to what a sculptress does in molding a statue out of formless clay, or a musician who forms lovely music from random notes and precise intervals of silence. You will also learn to explore ideas, to pay close attention to what others in small groups say and do and to engage your feelings with emotional agility.

If you are not sure it's for you, visit a theater or school where improv classes are held and watch students perform after just a few hours of training. You'll be amazed - and motivated to be part of an art form for those who seek to thrive and flourish.

17. LET CHARMING AND LIKABLE BE YOUR PERSONALITY HOMEPAGE

Guard against the all-too-human tendency to sling poo - that is, to be a *slingpoo.*

A *slingpoo* is one who continually and gratuitously denigrates, maligns or otherwise besmirches the reputation, physical appearance, ideas or accomplishments of others. Of course, this is not something unique to seniors, but seniors often are accused of being negative. Besides, negative people often grow up to become seniors. So, whether it's just to boost the image of elders, or to become more fun to be around, cease and desist in *slingpoo-ing*, if so tempted. Now's a good time to fine-tune your charming and likable personality. (The neologism credit in this case goes to Brenda J. Gannam, as published in the always delightful *AWADmail*, Issue 839, July 29, 2018.)

As part of your charm and likability, guard against inadvertently undermining the accomplishments or sources of pride others may express. There is a neologism for this, too, thanks to Margaret Stein of Omaha, NE. (A.Word.A.Day *AWADmail* Issue 820, March 18, 2018.) It's called a *toptale*. A *toptale* is one who turns conversations into competitions by one-upping the speaker. For instance, if you manage to complete your first triathlon without drowning, crashing on the bike or walking the entire run, he'll mention winning the *First Timers* division in his initial outing. Or, if you did a sprint triathlon, he tells you about his Ironman.

Ms. Stein offered these examples of a toptale:

> *If you ruined your suit in the thunderstorm, his basement was flooded.*

> *If you saw Lin-Manuel Miranda on Broadway, he won VIP tickets and met him backstage.*

> *If your aunt just peacefully passed away, his died last week by spontaneous combustion.*

61

As with *slingpoo-ing*, relentless and insufferable *toptale-ing* has no place in your charming and likable persona.

18. INFLUENCE AND DAZZLE

Dale Carnegie influenced a lot of people.

His tips for success, both social and financial, put forward in 1936 in *How to Win Friends and Influence People,* focused on showing a genuine interest in other people. Carnegie's recommendations were simple enough but underappreciated then as now - smile a lot, remember names, be a good listener, address topics others care about, make everyone feel important - and perform all these and other tips with sincerely.

All were and remain keys to guiding others to feel important, respected and appreciated. The challenge was developing the skills and readiness to manifest these traits sincerely.

All these qualities are invaluable in later life as well. Be alert to old people stereotypes - make a point not to appear cranky, self-centered, dismissive, cantankerous or forgetful - unless doing so might, on rare occasions, give you some advantage! (While feigning memory loss can be useful, it must not be overdone, less your children might be tempted to hide your car keys.)

Be wary of expectations some might harbor about senior citizens. While it must be admitted that a few mature folks can be annoying, so, too, are many young and middle-age people. Boorish and off-putting behaviors are observed in all age groups.

Basically, a good way to win friends and influence people during your senior years is to do the unexpected, such as listening to the opinions of others - and showing respect for all voices.

19. GIVE HOMAGE TO MARCEL PROUST — REMEMBER FRIENDS PAST

Nurture valued friendships, especially if they're nearly as old as you are.

Make regular efforts to stay in touch with those who were close over the years, from your school days, early career stages and similar good and/or memorable times. Later life presents new difficulties; getting by with a little help from friends can mean a lot.

One of the greatest of novels contained this theme. You may not know French, but you've probably seen the famous phrase, *À la recherche du temps perdu* — generally translated as *Remembrance of things past*. Proust's epic novel *Remembrance of*

Things Past consists of seven volumes written between 1909 and his death in 1922. The work consists of childhood recollections and memorable experiences into adulthood in early 20th-century aristocratic France, much of which reflects the loss of time and lack of meaning to the world.

Connections take more effort as one ages - people move, lose touch and don't get around much anymore. Familiar faces with whom you have shared experiences matter. To all, offer tender words and, every now and then, express in your own fashion an acknowledgment of the bond you share.

Sharon Roggenbuck gives homage to this idea, as follows:

> *Friendships are very dear to me, and I make every effort to hang on to them. I have one dear friend from the 9th grade. We see each other from time to time. I also stay in touch with my first boyfriend - from high school. Others in my circle have been there for over 60 years. We connect through letters, birthday cards, e-mails, phone calls and Facebook. From time to time I take trips to see friends. The older I get, the more important it is to maintain these friendships.*

In a speech entitled, *The Foundations of Faith*, Ingersoll suggested that we:

Cultivate the mind, become familiar with the mighty
thoughts that genius has expressed, the noble deeds of all the
world;
Cultivate courage and cheerfulness,
Fill life with the splendor of generous acts, the warmth of
loving words;
Discard error, destroy prejudice and receive new truths with
gladness;
Cultivate hope, see the calm beyond the storm, the dawn
beyond the night.

20. BE GRATEFUL

Gratitude doesn't change the scenery. It merely washes clean
the glass you look through so you can clearly see the colors.
Richelle E. Goodrich

Resolve to develop a habit of waking up with an attitude of
gratitude. As soon as you open your eyes and sort things out
(e.g., where you are and how you got there), smile and
exclaim a few words suitable to the occasion. An example
might be something along these lines:

Holy cow! I'm still alive. I'm going to have some fun today!
Everything's going to be all right! I am so grateful to the
universe for my good fortune.

You can come up with a more personal, satisfying exclamation, no doubt.

The reasons for gratitude are endless, beyond being alive. Chances are, you have a roof over your head, you don't struggle to get enough to eat and your basic needs are comfortably met. No cause for pessimism in any of that.

Be creative in your thoughts about gratitude. For instance, you might decide to be thankful that it's the 21st century, not some grim period and/or place in history, such as during the 700 years when Pope Paul III's Holy Office of the Universal Inquisition went on a tear to *maintain and defend the integrity of the faith and proscribe errors and false doctrines*. As one partial to a few errors and false doctrines myself, (Don), I'm grateful that I live in a time and place where I can't be found guilty of riding a bicycle on a Sunday, thereby finding myself chained upside down, nekked, in a dungeon, attended by holier-than-thou maniacal sadists. Now that's something to be grateful about.

Another way of commemorating this positive attitude, besides the personal felt appreciation for your own good fortune, is to be of service to others. Consider reaching out to extend charity, knowledge and/or assistance in your special ways to someone or many others. Susan Bradley-Cox loved the sport of triathlon, and many other sports she enjoyed growing up, and knew that others would enjoy such activities, as well, if given a helping hand getting started. As a result, she now devotes considerable time to volunteer coaching in several disciplines, including cheerleading and gymnastics, sports in which she excelled as a young girl. Of note - Susan organized a triathlon nearly two decades ago in order to raise funds for eye research - and that event is now in its 17th year. Can you guess for whom the USAT sanctioned *Susan Bradley-Cox Tri for Sight* is named?

Bottom line - don't take your good fortune and bright future for granted. Billions of people do not have luxuries or much of a life at all. Few in the long arc of human history could imagine the good fortune that you enjoy. Anu Garg captured this idea without going back centuries to express some of the wonders of contemporary life relative to decades ago when participants in this project were schoolchildren:

> *Imagine just 50 years ago, you met someone who told you that in the future you'd be carrying a radio, a television, a record player, a calculator, a clock, a camera, a photo album, a library, not to mention a telephone, with you every day, everywhere. And all this would nicely fit in your pocket. (Source: A.Word.A.Day with Anu Garg, Wordsmith.org, January 28, 2018.)*

Which brings to mind Winston Allen's advice about gratitude:

Be sure to acknowledge and thank the person/persons who have helped you significantly in attaining your successes before you, or they, pass on. I have done this by letter and in person and it made me feel good about myself knowing I would have regretted it if I didn't.

Yes, be grateful and don't be shy about showing it. Optimistic, grateful people are happier and healthier people and they usually share their good fortune with others!

21. PONDER THE POSSIBILITIES

There are all kinds of prospects and potentials within your capability - find a few and have at them.

Find ways to sustain an active interest in as many little things as possible, provided they entertain, amuse and do no harm. This in no way interferes with the select number of larger goals and purposes about which you are already passionate. Having interesting things to do, pursuits small and large, helps the blood get where it needs to go and lubricates parts (metaphorically speaking) that animate your days.

Pay attention to your stress level when stepping out and trying new tricks—remember that the goal is not to avoid stress—it's to sustain interests while maintaining peace of mind, that is, a placid state of centeredness.

Remember this goal when venturing beyond your comfort zone. Know that attitude is almost everything, regrets count for little and it's best not to look back—*something might be gaining on you.* (Thanks, Satchel.)

Consider Lockett Wood's attitude:

> *At 80, I'm still making 10-year plans - and hope to be here to see them achieved. I have plans for improved business activities and for new adventures, such as flying a small airplane, skydiving, visiting American Samoa and biking the nation's national parks.*

When you wake, ask yourself, *what fun things shall I do first today?* Nothing dramatic is necessary - pick up a book or newspaper to read with breakfast, walk the dog, do a dance and sing along to a stirring tune (e.g., *You Can't Always Get What You Want*). Think of a few things you've never done that just might be worth considering before it's too late. Who knows? *If you try sometimes you might find you get what you need.*

22. WHAT A SPECIMEN THOU ART

Don't hide your dynamism. This is no time for false (or even true) modesty. It's time to appreciate the fact that (in some ways), you are a mighty specimen of your species.

Really, all things considered, you have reason to be proud. And you should feel good about yourself, in good measure because a healthy self-concept adds exuberance and all that comes with it. Consider the immortal words of Stuart Smalley and proclaim, to yourself, with chin up and hands on hips when no one's around,

> *I'm good enough, I'm smart enough and doggone it, people like me!*

Treat yourself in a first-class manner, whenever affordable. Go forth with shoulders back. Look on the bright side of life, groom carefully and be your natural dynamic self. Bring into sharp focus in your own mind the critical point that good posture matters. Jack has long observed that some of the older men and women at his gym needlessly walk slowly, so prodigiously pokey they appear to be shuffling. Jack wonders, *why do this if it can be helped? Why let one's posture surrender to gravity without resistance?*

Seemingly aimless plodding along invites poor posture and a host of other negative signals to others, as well as adversely affecting oneself.

Make no mistake about it, the tendency to slow down comes with the territory in *Longevity-land*. Thus, Jack reminds himself to make a point of striding with confidence, knowing that doing so serves his own wellbeing by making him feel and look better.

Being well maintained physically and looking good will make you feel better, too. Old age is no time for self-doubt. Celebrate your wonderfulness before it's too late - there's no assurance others will do so when you're gone and, besides, even if they do, you won't know about it.

23. HAVE SOMETHING SPECIAL ON THE HORIZON

We all live under the same sky, but we don't all have the same horizon. Konrad Adenauer

Plan an event or adventure a few months to a year ahead. Such a plan need not and should not be an absolute, unmodifiable commitment, such as the determination you have for living a healthful, enjoyable and meaningful life, as long as possible. Rather, the idea of one or more special future events, such as a cruise, an organized bike tour in an

71

unfamiliar city, a night at the opera, a concert featuring a favorite artist - whatever meets your fancy, adds luster to the future. It's good to have something worthy of eager anticipation, a highlight to come of value.

An anticipated event or activity is an attractive way to enhance interest in moving ahead, avoiding excessive focus on the here and now that may, at times, seem dull, gray and boring. Perhaps something as simple as plans to be somewhere strange or off-the-beaten path in the not-too-distant future.

Something special on the horizon also means you have a positive, attractive reason to be around in a few months or next year. Therefore, you will be more likely to look after yourself. Include in the menu of possibilities consideration of a trip to see family members, a long-lost friend or an intriguing new place. For our *Not Dead Yet* set, being a triathlete usually entails travel to interesting places, in addition to the excitement of racing. Having something new and different coming up adds a small measure of zest and anticipation.

24. PERFORM A GOOD-HUMORED SECULAR EXORCISM

Consider this tip for one or more miscreants and evildoers from your past who might be suitable as foils for entertaining, theatrical-like fun, namely, the casting out of demons.

Just know that this is all in good fun—we don't want anyone being serious about demons or mythological evil spirits, trolls, ogres, vampires, ghosts or whatever rumored to go bump in the night, thereby frightening little children and primitive peoples.

A little homemade theater can serve for gaiety, followed by a period of serenity and peace. Nearly everyone who has lived past middle age has suitable candidates for such an exercise in mental cleansing. You really can't live a long life without encountering vexatious, dishonest, mean-spirited and otherwise villainous and even nefarious individuals. A few characters over the years have no doubt wronged you - and they deserve retribution, condemnation, a tongue-lashing or, in some cases, long prison sentences. But, such sweet comeuppances Hollywood-style are unlikely, expensive, possibly illegal, time-consuming and, more than not, unsuccessful.

But play-acting and having a good hoot while engaging in a little silliness among friends and fans of your eccentricity can be quite satisfying. Why carry around lingering feelings of anger, resentment, stress or hostility when you can have fun working out old grudges harmlessly? Holding ill feelings is like taking poison and expecting someone else to die. Let it all go—time is of the essence and life is always too short to be vexed some, most or all the time.

So, create an exorcism ceremony and have a ball cleansing your soul, mind or heart. For instance, maybe you could, in an environmentally friendly way, put the names of varied malefactors in a small pile and set it ablaze while wearing a silly witch doctor-like outfit and mumbling a chant, speaking in tongues. Or, if you have enough enemies, make a giant bonfire and torch it, creating your own *Burning Man* extravaganza. (Please check with your fire department before going through with this idea.) Play some music, perform a dance, make a toast or give a speech. Consider enlisting a colorful celebrity or pompous politician in your theatrical casting out of an evil spirit.

While irreverent about the ritual, know that the act has a meaningful purpose—it's to rid your awareness of those you would have preferred, in hindsight, had never made it there in the first place. Few of us cannot recall a few such bad actors.

Chapter Four

Athleticism Dimension: Tips for Sound Nutrition and Vigorous
Daily Exercise

25. ALL TIPS ARE EQUAL BUT THIS ONE'S MORE EQUAL

Vigorous daily exercise and nutritious, delicious and only
occasionally pernicious meals are a foundation for successful
aging.

Exercise and a sound diet are so interrelated that they should
be treated as a single topic, which is how we address this
dimension of successful aging. Aging is inexorable, however,
the nature, extent and timing of its effects vary as a
consequence of lifestyle, especially the quality of exercise and
diet habits over time. A New Scientist report found overeating
a bigger global health problem than lack of food. (Source:
Jessica Hamzelou, *Overeating Now Bigger Global Problem Than
Lack Of Food,* Home News, December 13, 2012.)

The data are startling - the World Health Organization
(WHO) reports that worldwide obesity has nearly tripled
since 1975 and that 52% of adults are overweight or obese. In
America, these figures are surely much higher. WHO also
notes that obesity is preventable.

Nearly everyone knows that exercise and food choices are critical factors affecting how we age, but making sound choices day after day, for years and years, is regarded as too much trouble by most Americans. Those without a deeply held commitment to exercise and sound diet will not age successfully.

Yet, now that you are getting up in years, it's more important than ever to overcome obstacles to managing both priorities. To succeed at aging, a few prerequisite steps can be immensely helpful:

1. Find a qualified coach/mentor to guide your initial efforts.
2. Do what you can to be ensconced within a supportive culture that reinforces healthy food choices, ensuring that you ingest the kind of nutrients you need for optimal functioning without having to go out of your way or struggle mightily to do so. This is difficult even with the best of intentions if this requires separation from long familiar customs and habits inimical to wellbeing.
3. Identify and eliminate as many obstacles and barriers as possible (environmental and otherwise) that compromise sound exercise and dining choices.

The principal options are starkly different now—you can either take (or remain on) the path that leads to thriving and flourishing—or succumb much sooner to the frailties associated with old age. Bodies are affected by gravity and devolution much faster if left to decay from inattention and neglect.

Want to guess what percentage of middle-aged and older adults in the Western world exercise at even a minimal level? For those over 65, the consensus answer among exercise scientists is about 10%! One recent study of older men and women revealed that those who exercised regularly enjoyed less stress and illnesses and better reflexes, memories, balance and metabolic profiles. How much better? Hold your hat - their wellbeing levels were closer to 30-year-olds than to their sedentary peers. (Source: Ross D. Pollock et. al., *An investigation Into the Relationship Between Age and Physiological Function in Highly Active Older Adults,* The Journal of Physiology, January 2015.)

A follow-up study focused on muscles and T cells, which are key infection-fighting components of the immune system. The findings gave further support for the potent value of nature's greatest drug - regular exercise. The 75+ exercisers were healthier and biologically much younger than expected for men and women of their chronological years.

Biological age, it's clear, is more consequential than actual age and, unlike the latter, is modifiable with health-enhancing initiatives. The tip in this case is self-evident - get moving and eat wisely. Be athletic, even if you never compete. Some exercise is better than none, but don't settle for the mediocrity of dabbling workouts like a fitness dilettante.

26. DON'T CALL IT QUITS TOO SOON

Aging well is relative, like nearly everything else.

Winston Allen said, *I've heard athletes say, I want to quit while I'm on top,* or *I have too much respect for the sport to perform at less than my optimal level.* Winston suggests that you not believe this for a minute. The deeper motivation, probably not even a conscious one, is that they think the sport won't be fun anymore. Their standard of performance has diminished. That's how most of us once felt as we got older and slowed down. It was more fun being fast and winning races, crowds cheering and people looking at you in awe. (OK, maybe it wasn't quite like that, but you get the idea—you were pretty good.)

Fortunately, most of us get over this bit of irrationality, and for good reason—the other guys and gals are in the same boat—they're aging, too. The good news is you no longer need to be so darn speedy, everyone else in your division or age cohort is slowing, many more so than you, especially if you follow the *Not Dead Yet* vigorous lifestyle tips for vitality and maximal flourishing, and they don't.

If you enjoy your sport, or avocation/activity of any kind but feel you can no longer do the things that were once a proverbial piece of cake, don't fret about it. Be rational—you won't have any need to swallow or otherwise incur damage to your pride if you just accept that you're human and getting slower is part of the deal. Despite slowing, most activities will still provide as much benefit and enjoyment as earlier in life, though this may not apply for professional athletes, like 41-year-old NFL superstar Tom Brady or the legendary Leroy *Satchel* Paige (July 7, 1906 – June 8, 1982), who played until he was 59 years, 351 days old. A perennial if there ever was one.

You don't have to be the best. Just be the best that you can be, and sometimes you might still be the best in your group.

Whenever asked how he did in a race, one of us (Don), says he won his division. If curiosity does lure the questioner to the obvious follow-up query (i.e., *What division might that be?),* Don prods the mark by adding that he's won his division in every race he's done for the past 20 years. This seldom fails to impress or inspire skepticism, but if the victim of Don's trickery still does not ask the obvious follow-up question, Don adds, *can you guess my division?* No one ever has done so correctly, so Don tells him what it is, namely *the Grandmaster male division for those who are 6'3' and 170 pounds, right-handed with blue eyes, live in Florida, enjoy a REAL wellness lifestyle and have an odd sense of humor*. After a pause for guffaws and such, Don adds the punch line: *If you put yourself in the right division, you can win, too*. That, Don believes, is the key to thriving and flourishing at all stages of life — to create your own division, one that includes following a REAL wellness lifestyle.

Winston Allen claims he can relate to the value of this tip. He held the Hawaiian Ironman swim record for four years in the 65-69 age group. Since then, he's had both knees replaced, and the added weight causes his lower body to sink a good bit. Now he considers himself a back-of-the-pack swimmer and, alas, his run has been reduced almost to a walk. Regardless of all that, and despite being on the cusp of 90, Winston still competes and, more important, still enjoys the sport of triathlon.

27. EAT WELL

A sound diet, weighted in whole grains, fruits, vegetables and nuts will help you look your best and stay well.

Most people follow a diet pattern more or less consistent with whatever was served on tables set by their parents and caregivers in their first decades. Our initial acculturation is how we chose the language we speak, the loyalties we adopted and the religious belief systems we embraced as our own. As the traditional Gospel song dating from 1873 goes,

Give me that old time religion
It was good for my old mother
It was good for my old father
And it's good enough for me.

This is arguably not the most enlightened way to choose a worldview, but it's the only and most natural way for all. However, early childhood habits may not stand the test of time as we grow, learn and fine-tune choices in accord with our own experiences. It's clearly a good idea to update food preferences and diet patterns based upon discoveries over time that enable people to maximize both enjoyment and health status by making informed food choices.

Obtain basic information about nutritional dining by relying on reputable experts, and on organizations not selling food products, such as weight loss or other diet books. Choices we make on our own, informed by varied and well-vetted sources, are usually more reliable than those to which we were acclimated before we were mature and informed sufficiently to choose for ourselves.

You're a big boy or a grown woman now, and *the future lies ahead,* as comedian Pat Paulsen often observed. Time now to free yourself from a diet pattern that may not have been quite right for you, either health-wise or for weight-management purposes. Look for a pattern of dining that, over time, will taste just as good if not better than the one you first adopted. Such is likely to render more satisfying outcomes for your wellbeing and appearance.

There is no shortage of both genuine and bogus experts with diet plans, cookbooks and nutrition studies and theories. It's between hard to impossible to be certain your current approach is the best food plan. Well-meaning friends and money-grubbing mountebanks galore are willing and anxious to offer their food plan, but many have a conflict of interest. That is, their interests (profit) and yours (good health) may not align.

How can you know whom to trust, whose advice is sound and what patterns will work best? There is no sure fire, guaranteed way, sorry to say. However, there are things you can do to improve your chances. Familiarize yourself with alternatives, look closely at evidence claims, seek advice from reputable authorities and try varied approaches. Don't settle on a favorite approach prematurely. Stay open-minded while you assess what diet plan seems to make the most sense for you in that it provides the best results.

28. IS IT TOO LATE?

It's probably not too late to begin exercise and diet reforms.

Naturally, many do wait too long and never have a chance to get started. For example, when medical emergency terms like *red alert, all hands-on deck* or *extreme unction* are being bandied about, it might be too late to get started. During most of life, however, improvements are possible, usually of the dramatic kind. Get started today, slowly and easily, then little by little and bit by bit, pick up the pace. Do a little more each day. At least 50% of our triathlon champions took up the sport in their 50s or even later. A few were not even athletes when they started feeling old and decided it was time to shape up and fly right! This was one of our surprising discoveries while reading the author bios, which you can view in the Appendix.

Whether the impetus or epiphany was a mirror, a shortness of breath, a concerned mate, a doctor or a medical scare, deciding it was time to start moving was crucial to the transformations of our champions who reported a late start on exercise. Just look how they evolved - from couch potatoes to champion triathletes.

Take Roger Brockenbrough, for example. Roger agrees that it's never too late. With some prodding from his son John, he became interested in fitness and triathlons when in his early

50s. Prior athleticism was limited to pick-up games as a kid and touch football. Easing into it gradually, he lost 20 pounds over the first year of consistent vigorous exercise - and lowered his resting heart rate about 20 points. To his surprise, he found he had a talent for running, which he built upon while also embracing swimming and biking. The challenge to improve his performance served to inspire an aggressive pursuit of triathlon, which he's been doing for 30-some years.

Swimming was Roger's greatest challenge at first. He learned to swim the hard (not recommended) way at a Boy Scout camp when over-exuberant (and no doubt unsupervised) staffers threw him in a river. He survived that but developed a fear of water that had to be overcome. Little could he have imagined at the time of the *swim or sink* lesson that he would eventually do nine 2.4-mile swims as part of Ironman distance races. Roger did his first Ironman at age 61. At that time, he still had a measure of anxiety about the swim, especially one offering such a daunting distance challenge. Worries began days before the race when he looked out at the course and could barely see the turn-around marker. He thought, *OMG, what have I gotten myself into?* For a moment, he reconsidered the whole idea. Fortunately, this disquiet was quickly overcome. And well that it was, for swim conditions on race day were daunting. However, Roger forged ahead, literally taking the plunge into the misty deep. Battered by waves, colliding with other competitors in turbulent waters and taking in more seawater than could have been good for his health or state of mind, he again revisited the thought of quitting, but banished the idea once more. Thus, despite breast stroking and heaving during the final 200 yards, he made it in. The swim accomplished, his prospects improved during the bike and run. Roger ended up winning his age group! Lesson learned: Do all you can before retiring prematurely, as a general rule.

By the way, Roger has had many additional successes since that first Ironman, winning national and world triathlon titles and being inducted into the USAT Hall of Fame on January 16, 2016.

So, never mind that Chinese expression about a journey of a thousand miles commencing with a first step. This isn't about a thousand miles or making a late-in-life transition into becoming a triathlete. It is, however, about a more important mission - taking steps to shape the quality of the rest of your life. If not already on your way to or established with a REAL wellness lifestyle, get started. Today!

While aging can't be prevented, decay can be avoided or, if necessary, treated and eliminated by prudent actions on your part.

The complexity of your body makes the contemporary world wide web seem as simple as Guglielmo Marconi's 1895 radio signaling system. Your body has billions of cells; chemical messages travel throughout the body via the nervous and circulatory systems. Trillions of internal signals are continually interacting via nerve connections, hormonal receptors and the bloodstream communicating with all tissues in the body.

Don't fret about something you can't prevent (i.e., aging); instead, do something every day (exercise and eat well) that promotes vitality despite aging declines.

We want you to be a lifestyle artist, a model of wise living. You can do this not with heroic physical efforts but with moderate exercises, such as daily walks. Eat well and get eight to nine hours of sleep on average. Nearly everyone knows what's entailed in practicing elementary good health habits, especially regular vigorous exercise. The trick is getting started and staying at it long enough to experience the satisfactions that will naturally motivate you to make exercise a pleasurable part of every day.

29. JOIN A WELL-EQUIPPED CLUB

In time, you will lose a bit of speed, endurance will diminish and recovery from exertions will take longer. Injuries might also become more frequent, breakdowns more common and healing will be slower. However, there are actions that can delay these annoyances.

Regular gym workouts will help, as will exertions of core and leg muscles. Get creative about everyday balance actions, such as putting socks on and removing them while standing up. (If you think that's easy, give it a try. It will seem almost impossible at first but, after a few ungainly attempts, you will master this curious ability.) One of our champions claims he enters his bed every night with a flying leap. (We're skeptical about this claim so we don't recommend it.)

Kidding aside, balance, flexibility and strength are valuable additions to the cardio work you can do on your own, with coaching or in classes at nearly all gyms. Think of the passage of time as a form of crossing an unknown and difficult creek or stream. For most of the crossing, things have gone reasonably well and much progress has been made. Now, however, you're nearly there, that is, on the other side. The water seems deeper, moves faster and the bottom is rocky, making footholds uncertain. Balance has become much harder. There is no way back.

As a senior, that somewhat describes the fix you're in. You're not stuck in a creek, stream or river, so you can work on skills that need sharpening, balance among them. Practice simple agility moves that help muscles adapt and your reflexes remain tuned.

Knowing how important fitness is, Sharon Roggenbuck teaches a strength and stretching class. Sharon says,

> *My emphasis is on gaining and maintaining strength for everyday activities, practicing posture, stretching and balance work (more important as we age). These components help the aging body look and feel stronger.*

Gyms come in many forms and cater to different athletic interests with price structures from bare bones to haute couture. Visit several close to your home or place of work.

There is one important exercise that you can obtain in a typical gym not otherwise available in the great outdoors – strength training. You can, with free weights, reinvigorate your neurotransmitters, which coordinate balance, thereby preventing deterioration over time. Alas, this does not happen with endurance exercise, which primarily adds to the staying power of muscles. Strength training builds the power in muscles needed to coordinate movements with grace, balance and efficiency. Strength training, in short, enables you to recruit maximum nerve cells so that muscles most effectively coordinate between brain and the rest of body. Strength training is a vital factor in strengthened nerve connections with stronger tendons, ligaments and joints. Would you be surprised to learn that falls are *the* leading cause of fatal and nonfatal injuries among older adults? According to *New York Times* health columnist Jane E. Brody, *every 19 minutes in this country, an older person dies from a fall.* (Source: Jane E. Brody, *Falls Can Kill You. Here's How to Minimize the Risk,* New York Times, February 25, 2019.) Basically, you are less likely to fall from stumbling on a crack in a sidewalk because your recovery reflexes will be faster, but if you do lose your balance and fall from such a misstep, you are likely to incur less damage from doing so.

Weight lifting is hard and requires more skill and practice than using machines. Hire a coach, learn to lift properly but don't overdo it in early sessions. This form of exercise might be the best of all reasons for belonging to a gym. Do strength training twice a week for at least 30 minutes. It's not easy (it can and will be an ordeal until you learn to appreciate the positive effects); if all the discipline required to follow REAL wellness lifestyles were easy, everyone would look great and thrive throughout their senior years. We know that's not the case in America or anywhere else.

30. TREAT YOURSELF TO REGULAR MASSAGES

Massage is the answer—who cares what the question is? Time spent getting a massage is never wasted. While aging can't be prevented, decay can be avoided or, if necessary, treated and eliminated by prudent actions on your part.

Regular massages are a good idea, rich with benefits for prevention and health enhancement. Having skin, muscles, tendons and ligaments rubbed, squeezed, manipulated and pressured speeds healing of minor injuries and adds resistance to looming problem areas. Sharon Roggenbuck treats herself to a monthly massage because she enjoys it and knows how beneficial it is.

Besides spas, massage services are popular in a range of settings, such as health and wellness centers, medical facilities, companies and even airports. Such therapies take many forms, such as Swedish (long strokes, kneading, deep circular movements, vibration and tapping), deep massage (slower, more-forceful strokes that target muscle and connective tissue), trigger point (tight muscle fibers) and more.

Many benefit claims are made to justify regular massages. This is not a science thoroughly researched by neutral parties. For one thing, variables are hard to control (e.g., who's doing the massage, the multiplicity of techniques or schools of massage etc.). Enthusiasts for massage claim that it reduces stress, speeds muscle recovery from vigorous exercise and mitigates a variety of medical issues, such as headaches, insomnia and joint pain.

Beyond the benefits real or imagined, it would be enough if massages simply led to good feelings all over and a sense of comfort, relaxation and connection.

31. GET IT DONE, BUT DON'T BE TYRANNICAL ABOUT IT

Seek a happy medium between faithfulness to a workout schedule and flexibility to adjust when conditions warrant. Weather is unpredictable, training partners do not always show up, special occasions require alterations in routines and energy levels vary - so be flexible about when, where and how to exercise. Established habits for doing things that matter are generally good and help you stay on track, but you still must retain the power to grant waivers to yourself when it serves, and to do so without guilt, remorse or hesitation. You are, after all, the maestro who alone orchestrates your workouts and overall fitness plan. The bottom line must be the ways and means that produce the best performance in terms of satisfactions. Who wants to have a schedule anyway? After decades of pursuing a career with demanding time constraints, most of us aren't anxious to imprison ourselves to inflexible routines. Schedules that enable you to prevent or at least restrain muscle losses that attend normal aging are vital and regularity is essential, but inflexibility is not necessary or desirable.

A fit body takes a lot of work; it requires determination over time to achieve and maintain. Those who did not enter later life fit will find it more challenging to achieve and maintain physical fitness. It can still be done and must be done to live well, enjoy and otherwise age successfully.

Our aging champions and millions of others manage to age and stay fit; all the former want you to do the same, despite the difficulties.

Dr. Bill Ziering recommends body movement, the opposite of the *prolonged rest* that physicians used to advise for aches and pains associated with aging and other agents of physical woe. He also favors half-hour brisk walks for combating negativity and one or more of the following as substitutes for an aspirin a day—aerobic and resistance training, swimming, yoga, Tai Chi, Pilates, Qigong, dancing, martial arts or whatever other activity can be managed that strengthens the body, boosts the immune system and lengthens those tell-tale telomeres.

Indubitable, undeniable and unimpeachable evidence supports the advice you have heard many times - a healthy lifestyle may prevent or at least postpone heart attacks, strokes, diabetes, arthritis and cancer. So how about it? If not already a devout adherent of the *exercise is good medicine* congregation, join the flock of Americans who are doing right by themselves, their families and their country, the latter since we can't afford the economy-wrecking costs of unnecessary but continually escalating medical conditions.

A gym will be invaluable for keeping aging at bay for longer periods of time, thus enabling an extended period of vitality. Physical fitness acts somewhat like sandbags in holding back rising floodwaters - it's not a permanent fix (there is none) but it delays and often prevents the predictable damages (frailties) of a rising tide of nature's troubles.

32. CHOOSE A FAVORITE DIET

There are endless varieties of diets, and nearly everyone has a favorite. We are no exception. The comments that follow are largely based on the preferences of the co-authors, with participant exceptions where noted. Everything mentioned in this tip, and all the others, was reviewed throughout the writing process by all participants, but that does not mean everyone signed a pledge of allegiance to all our opinions or took an oath to dine accordingly forevermore.

To commence our diet tip, a few facts are in order concerning the typical American diet—which is no conscious diet at all –

just eat whatever is served, available, affordable and/or tastes good.

Not coincidentally, about two-thirds of Americans die of cancer or heart disease. Both are linked to poor diet patterns over time, though not exclusively. These and other disorders have multiple causes, including not just food patterns but also genetics and environmental factors.

There are enough books heralding the best diet/weight loss and/or nutritional path to total wellbeing to fill a small public library, if not the Library of Congress.

There is little consensus on the best plan. The closest we have to a consensus national diet plan might be the *2015–2020 Dietary Guidelines* produced by the federal Office of Disease Prevention and Health Promotion. The guidelines provide five overarching principles and many recommendations for nutritional targets and dietary limits. All are designed to help Americans understand and follow a pattern that a wide range of experts recommend as a healthier diet pattern. However, food manufacturers, food producers and other special interest groups have an outside role in which parts of *the most current scientific evidence* are included. The sugar, dairy and beef industries, for instance, successfully lobby to limit advice inimical to their very popular products, despite evidence that many are somewhat between unhealthful and disastrous.

Diet books might do more harm than good; some eventually prove to be unhealthy, wacky and dangerous. We urge that you be conscientious, disciplined and choose wisely. Settle on a consumption pattern that will complement the other positive initiatives you follow to age successfully. Focus on the quality of food items, not the calories they contain.

Besides being conscientious about what you can, do what you can to promote, encourage and otherwise support food industry reform. A 2019 report based on three years of work by scientists from around the world projects dramatic changes in our food systems in the next 30 years. The study, described in the medical journal *Lancet*, calls for a *Great Food Transformation,* noting that meat-eating has *dire consequences for the planet.* The study authors recommend a largely plant-based diet. If this does not happen within 30-years-time, climate change and an increase in global population will bring about large-scale starvation. This scenario is based on projected side effects of food production, including greenhouse gases, water and crop use, more nitrogen and phosphorus from fertilizers and diminished biodiversity. In order to reduce meat and sugar consumption by 50%, a vegan diet is recommended. A similar study with comparable recommendations appeared in the journal *Nature,* October 2018.

A practical guide to healthy eating can be found in a popular book by Michael Greger, M.D., entitled, *How Not to Die*. This is based on thousands of his short instructional videos which, as he humorously put it, were *boiled down into this scant little 562-page book.*

Besides the meat, dairy and multiple other industries' opposition to plant-based whole foods diets, large numbers of well-informed expert individuals take strong exception to the studies cited above and the orientation of the authors to limit or refrain from animal products. At least one of our participants expressed an opposite take on an ideal diet. Here is physician and triathlon champion Dwight Lundell's take on the matter:

> *A critical component of being healthy and healthy aging is to remain disease free. Worldwide the most deaths are from obesity, diabetes and heart disease, all nutritional disorders. The dramatic rise in the incidence of obesity and diabetes coincides precisely with the issuance of the dietary guidelines for Americans, lots of whole grains, industrial seed oils, reduced animal fats, eggs, dairy and red meat.*

> *The result of these dietary recommendations is our current unprecedented levels of bad health. The EAT Lancet report referenced is more of the same, and the results will be the same, déjà vu all over again.*

The anti-red meat philosophy originates mostly in religion. Most popular in this country in the mid-1800s was the idea that red meat caused impure thoughts and animal propensities. John Harvey Kellogg assured us that his cornflakes would prevent masturbation. (It did not.)

Ellen G White, the co-founder of the Seventh-day Adventist church has had the most profound effect on promoting vegetarianism and anti-red meat worldwide. She may have been the first to say that red meat causes cancer.

If you are plant-based because of religion, I respect that. If you're plant-based for any reason, I respect that. I have no objection to eating plants. Just know that there is no credible evidence that red meat causes cancer or that saturated fat causes heart disease.

The key to being healthy and healthy aging is maintaining a normal blood sugar. Just like maintaining a normal oxygen level.

Carbohydrates are not bad. The overconsumption of them leads to elevated blood sugar, which leads to heart disease, diabetes and obesity, arthritis and premature aging. Several well-done experiments show that in normal, non-diabetic people, the typical American breakfast of cereal and skimmed milk causes a damaging rise of blood sugar levels.

97

The Blue Zone longevity study showed limiting total calories was the key to longevity in the five populations studied (though plant foods figured large in their diets).

My tip for healthy aging is to get adequate amounts of protein, natural fats and limit carbohydrate intake to maintain a normal blood sugar.

A glucometer is cheap at the local drugstore and is a great tool to make sure your blood sugar is normal. If you eat something and one hour later your blood sugar is over 140 don't eat that again!

Now I am going to grill and eat a delicious healthy steak with cheesy broccoli on the side and train hard tomorrow.

As noted previously, our 18 champions are not of a single mind on most topics. However, none question the value of regular vigorous exercise or the importance of lifestyle choices in advancing exuberance and preventing and/or delaying the onset of frailties.

While the co-authors do not wish to debate our champion participants when there is a disagreement, the suggestion that an *anti-red meat* orientation is religious in nature invites a notation. The non-religious co-authors favor a whole-foods, plant-based diet based upon personal preferences, which in their view is supported by an extensive body of evidence-based studies. Advocates for diets all make this claim, so the consumer must sort out what seems most persuasive among competing claims. Experts and followers of diets alike insist that science is on their side, just as warring nations usually claim that God is with us. Skeptics, including Abraham Lincoln during our Civil War, struggle to comprehend how God can back both antagonists.

The food industry will produce and promote healthier products when it's in their financial interest to do so. When the healthiest foods are prominently displayed in supermarkets, more people will select quality nutrients. Two things might move companies in this direction: 1) government supports, such as tax policies favoring high nutrient foods; and 2) changes in demands by better-educated consumers about the value and environmental advantages of whole foods, plant-based diets.

Such diets are not the easiest to follow. There are fewer vegan or vegetarian menu options in most restaurants. The diet requires more education and more attention to detail. Fortunately, simply increasing the balance of your meals with a wide range of vegetables, whole grains, nuts, seeds, legumes and fruits will, some of us believe, make a positive difference in the quality of your food pattern and consequent health status.

If you need to lose weight, this is the way to do it. Consider: You can eat these foods until you feel full and you don't need to count calories.

There is also a curious and serendipitous beneficial side effect of following a whole-foods, plant-based food pattern. Can you guess what that might be? It is that by filling up on delicious meals of a healthful nature, you diminish if not eliminate a lot of harmful foods. Sugary, fat-filled, salt-laden and other high-risk ingredients have little presence on healthy menus. The cravings for foods you know add little to nothing to overall wellbeing will not appeal quite as much, if at all, when you settle into a vegan-oriented diet, should you go that route.

Whatever you decide, stay flexible and be willing to adjust as new information becomes available. *Bonne chance, mon ami –* good luck, my friend!

33. EXPLORE SOME FORM OF MEDITATION

Like most Westerners, the participants involved in this book did not report being attracted to any of the varied forms of meditation. With one notable exception, the practice of contemplation, musing or engaging in one or more techniques for resting the mind or attaining a state of consciousness different from the normal waking state seems not to be a high priority, or priority at all.

Well, thanks to famed neuroscientist, philosopher and best-selling author Sam Harris and his *Making Sense* (formerly *Waking Up*) podcast, co-author, Jack began to take an interest in meditation and has had something of an epiphany about the practice. Jack noted that many guests on Sam's podcasts are practitioners of meditation, and Sam himself is an eloquent enthusiast about it. One guest, Yuval Noah Harari, the author of the best-seller *Sapiens: A Brief History of Humankind* caught Jack's attention. Dr. Harari spends two months each year at a meditation retreat and he attributes his success in good measure to his immersion in the art.

As a result, when a guided meditation app was offered by Sam Harris, Jack signed up and gave it a try. Three months and almost 50 meditation sessions later, Jack reports that this mental tool has helped him strengthen his focus, reduce distractions and disengage from unnecessary and unhelpful thoughts. What's more, the benefits of meditating appear to align with the mental needs and challenges associated with aging.

Jack notes that meditation is not a one-shot deal. It takes continuous practice, much like going to a gym and making the most of every visit. Jack meditates two or three times weekly, and reports that it, too, like swimming, running and biking, takes discipline and work. Without patience, the benefits can easily slip away.

34. SLOW DOWN, BE CALM, CHEW THOROUGHLY

It sounds easy, but not many take their meals in this manner. Whether you do so or not, consider learning the Heimlich maneuver. You might have an opportunity to come to the aid of a diner who failed to do one or more of this tip's simple dining practices. Choking is not uncommon.

Fine dining for taste and nutrient absorption entails mindfulness. Take your time and savor the moments, as well as the food and drink.

An Austrian study conducted between 1984 and 2001 urged thorough chewing to prevent the incidence of food/foreign body asphyxia. Semisolid foods lodged in the windpipe are the cause of many asphyxiations. You can't always count on someone ready and able to execute the Heimlich maneuver. This first-aid procedure for dislodging an obstruction from a windpipe by exerting a sudden, strong pressure applied on the abdomen between the navel and the rib cage has saved lives, but as noted, a skilled bystander is not always on the scene. In addition to being conscious about chewing thoroughly, there is one other element of this tip - learn to do the Heimlich maneuver so you can be the savior of someone who did not read this tip or otherwise learn this procedure.

Don once benefited from this maneuver. He was the speaker at a conference at The College of William and Mary in Williamsburg, VA in 1998. While chatting with dignitaries at the head table and simultaneously devouring a salad, Don felt a partial blockage in his windpipe. Not wanting to make a scene that might diminish his dignity, such as it was, he excused himself with the ill-conceived idea of walking it off (or out) in the adjacent hallway, conveniently just steps from his table. Bad idea - suddenly, more than loss of dignity seemed a possibility. Struggling to breathe, Don burst through the kitchen doors while pointing to startled cooks and dishwashers, sending pantomimed *do the Heimlich* clues in a desperate (and undignified) form of charades.

At first, all he accomplished was to strike fear that a madman was in the kitchen, but soon enough one of the workers got the idea, as much from the color of Don's face and size of his eyeballs, and performed a single chest compression from behind, thereby saving the conference leaders the inconvenience of having to find another speaker.
The moral of this story—forget about dignity—no one should ever suffer death by lettuce. Learn the Heimlich but if, for some reason, you never do, give it the old college try if you see someone out of breath, pointing to his throat and making

hugging gestures with his arms. The life you save may be some cockamamy with more dignity than common sense.

35. STAND TALL, CHIN UP, KEEP SHOULDERS BACK

Good posture in later life is no longer automatic or effortless--remind yourself to check whether you are standing erect and, if not, snap to attention. You want to appear impressive and staunch, not subdued and irresolute. With good posture, you'll feel stronger and look younger.

Winston Allen offers some invaluable advice on this tip:

> *As we age, we unconsciously start bending over when we walk, fail to pick our feet up and begin shuffling. This leads to falls, especially when encountering throw rugs, bath mats or uneven sidewalks and the like. So, walk straight and lift your feet - put some extra effort into it. No shuffling. I've noticed that walking erect automatically enables a higher stride level.*

If you have occasional lower back pain upon arising each morning, consider a daily ritual that Don finds the next-best thing to a quick fix. Lie down on your back on a hard surface, such as wood flooring. Gently, as mild pain permits, allow your spine to relax with full contact against the hard surface. If this is initially uncomfortable or even painful, know that this is a sure-sign that you need this exercise. Relax as much as possible for about a minute. After just a few seconds, there should no longer be pain--just relief. Draw one leg at a time to your chest, then both legs at one time. Turn your legs to one side, then the other.

That's it. When you rise (gently and slowly), your back should feel much better. If not, then this exercise is not for you. Don says he can't function without it.

Our lawyers want us to cover our butts by adding a word of caution and language to protect ourselves against ambulance chasers or anyone looking to exploit the legal system, though we believe that while such legal counsel is probably necessary, it's too bad it has come to this. But, here goes:

Before you do the above described simple relaxation stretch or anything else described in this book that you would not do absent reading about it here, know that life is hazardous and everything you do, whether we recommend it or not, is risky. Proceed with your life at your own discretion. We are NOT responsible for your exercise or lack thereof. We offer our best advice, which we think is fantastic, but we offer no guarantees if you choose to follow it.

36. KNOW THE FACTS AND TRENDS OF AGING

No matter how you earned the opportunity to exist for a span anywhere near the once remarkable age of 75, let alone older, you're likely to have plenty of company, even if you should reach *centenarian-hood*.

Your chances of doing so continue to improve, especially if you have achieved the impressive *rank* of septuagenarian, octogenarian or nonagenarian. If that's the case, congratulations - you are a credit to your species.

Longevity boosting habits, such as ample exercise, better diets, safer sex practices, reductions in infant and early childhood mortality and satisfying social networks, are among the trends that lead experts to project big increases in longer life in coming decades. This fact has implications for economies, job markets, social welfare (e.g., pensions), medical systems and quality of life in all nations with high rates of aging populations.

If you're a part of this elite age cohort, familiarize yourself with the facts of population trends; you can be a resource, an expert for friends who might dread the change of later year. With facts at your disposal, you can explain the opportunities inherent in later stages of life, thereby providing encouragement and support.

Hall of Fame triathlete James Ward, who died at 83 training for his next triathlon, believed the mind is the key to aging well while remaining active. You can offer this kind of encouragement to folks who are approaching retirement as well as those already in a senior age group, not just about triathlons, but about thriving and flourishing late in life.

In Japan, there were 153 centenarians in 1965 when such records were first collected; today there are 67,824. World Bank data indicates that 27% of Japan's population is 65 or older. Less than 10 years ago, the percentage of individuals 65+ in Japan was only 11%. The global population of seniors over 60 was 382 million in 1980; in 2017, it was 962 million and by 2050 it will be 2.1 billion, assuming no man-made or other global catastrophes. One final statistic - according to the US Census Bureau, the number of U.S. centenarians is projected to increase from 86,248 to at least 600,000 by 2060. We're taking over, folks. Time for a centenarian president?

An aging society will spark many changes in the larger work and leisure cultures, such as extended retirement ages, the advent of mid-career breaks or workforce sabbaticals, flexible labor patterns, job sharing, support for recurrent education and/or retraining on demand for interested retirees.

Such projections suggest that perennials can be a resource for the young as well as the aged. Perhaps you can utilize data like these to encourage and guide elderly friends to take better care of themselves. After all, seniors may be around longer than they once expected. It is more important than ever to age well, to remain as vital as possible as the years and decades bring dramatic changes for individuals and societies.

While it is immensely rewarding, it's not easy being a triathlete, at any age, especially during the later years. This is true for those who invest their energies in all endurance sports. Since we focused on 75 plus triathletes, we'll use their sport to make a point about hard choices, faced daily. As the writer E.B. White noted in the late 1800s, though not with triathletes in mind: *If the world were merely seductive, that would be easy. If it were merely challenging, that would be no problem. But I arise in the morning torn between a desire to improve the world and a desire to enjoy the world. This makes it hard to plan the day.*

But, who's to say that setting off each day to labor in a water body, ride a bike or go for a run is not a meaningful way to improve the world? Being a triathlete is both challenging and seductive in good ways, for the choice to train and compete safeguards and improves one's physical and mental wellbeing, models the benefits of self-discipline for the young and readies the individual to do what he or she thinks must be done.

Too bad E.B. White wasn't a triathlete—our sport would have made it easier for the good fellow to plan the day.

Chapter Five

Liberty Dimension: Tips for Personal Freedoms That Enable
You to Realize Your Desires, Interests and Preferences

> *There is a word sweeter than mother, home or heaven; that
> word is liberty.* Matilda Joslyn Gage

37. EXTEND TO ALL THE RIGHTS YOU CLAIM FOR YOURSELF

Faith or reason, superstition or science - choose your
preference and give everyone else the same opportunity.

Be an evangelist for liberty. Ingersoll called liberty *the blossom
and fruit of justice, the perfume of mercy.* Stand up and speak out
for choice and for freedom, while granting others' rights,
beliefs and preferences you may not favor yourself. The latter
suggests that you abide with tolerance even beliefs you find
objectionable. Say your piece and then move on - converts to
an opposing point of view are rarely instantaneous. Even if
you believe strongly in X, consider granting true believers in
Y space to think as they like. Perhaps, in earlier times, you
found meaning in advancing viewpoints about life's
persistent questions, but after doing so it's well to move on if
differences vex or otherwise perturb your companions.

Of course, if you're asked what you think, don't hesitate to lavish interested parties with the details of your amazing insights on certain topics, such as, say, religion, politics and/or sex, not necessarily in that order. But only if asked or otherwise invited. Consider what Albert Einstein had to say on this matter:

> *Unthinking respect for authority is the greatest enemy of truth.*

If not the greatest enemy, such unfettered respect is certainly no friend of freedom. This matters as much as ever, probably more so, in later years of life. At this stage, every opportunity should be seized to make room for unfettered positive thinking and good vibrations. As the great debunker James Randi has observed, *those who believe without reason cannot be convinced by reason.*

38. COMPLAINING IS MENTAL JUNKFOOD - FIND ALTERNATIVES

Stalks of roses are covered with thorns, but bouquets of roses are valued for the beauty and aromas of the flowers, never the thorns. Consider communicating in ways that attract, and as little as possible, repel.

Some sources credit Abraham Lincoln with coining the expression, *you can complain because roses have thorns, or you can rejoice because thorns have roses*, but at least half a dozen other possible authors of this bon mot surface when seeking the original author, including Ziggy, a cartoon character.

No matter - whoever said it knew that complaints often do more harm than good. Better to look for more creative ways to negotiate to right a wrong or otherwise get what you want.

Free yourself from the stress and negativity of complaining to the extent you can manage to do so. Complaints are akin to thorns in that they are irritants, and they often hurt, both the one doing the complaining and, naturally, the one on the receiving end. There are often more deliberative, liberating and intelligent ways to artfully address dissatisfactions, which represent more the rosebud approach.

Fortunate folks discover early in life that complaining or acting the victim, whining, blaming or excusing rarely gets you closer to goals or dreams, election to high office or named Mr./Ms. Popularity. Abandon tendencies toward righteous indignation, outrage or being quick to take umbrage, even if the slight, injury or offense might be consequential. You deserve to be treated better, more honestly or whatever, but it's wise not to give the impression that your complaint implies the other is a miscreant.

Come to think of it, why do so many complain so much?

One reason is to get action of some kind that rights a perceived wrong, that achieves a measure of justice, real or imagined. Another is to relieve stress. While on occasions, complaints make things a little better, more often, complaints . have adverse consequences.

Every day there are obstacles, problems, frustrations or setbacks. What might you do, in lieu of complaining, that would protect and enhance your preference for exuberant living, personal freedoms, positive relationships and common decencies, with no complaining to interrupt all these good experiences?

First, recognize the fact that eliminating or even reducing complaints might make things simpler, pleasanter and/or more enjoyable. In addition, it might liberate you, set you free from certain vexations. That's a measure of personal freedom not to be undervalued.

Here are a few minor things you can do to create a less complaint-oriented mindset:

- Practice not doing it and reward yourself when you succeed. You have to practice, to get good at anything, so be patient through a period of trial and error.

- Minimize contact with chronic complainers.
- Recognize that becoming disinclined to complain will retrain your brain to offer up alternative responses to aggravations.
- Focus less on yourself and more on solutions to little vexations.

Benefits might include the following:

- You will be viewed as more interesting and enjoyable to be around. Nobody loves a whiner.
- You will be a better role model for others, young and old.
- You will think more creatively. It's so easy to complain, gripe and whine - but it's a dead-end neural pathway.

In summary, eliminating or reducing complaints is an antidote for negativity, should there be any in or around your person. Unlikely, of course.

39. CONTENTMENT - THE MENTAL EQUIVALENT OF FITNESS

Mental health is the first and last element of wellbeing, and probably the middle one, as well.

This is an ungainly, unscientific and made-up way of expressing what the World Psychiatric Association (WPA) elegantly proclaimed (though with many more words) as an advance toward a new definition of mental health:

> *Mental health is a dynamic state of internal equilibrium which enables individuals to use their abilities in harmony with universal values of society. Basic cognitive and social skills; ability to recognize, express and modulate one's own emotions, as well as empathize with others; flexibility and ability to cope with adverse life events and function in social roles; and harmonious relationship between body and mind represent important components of mental health which contribute, to varying degrees, to the state of internal equilibrium.* (Source: *Toward a New Definition of Mental Health*, Journal of the World Psychiatry Association, June 14, 2015, pp. 231–233.)

Thus, mental fitness not only complements but probably enables physical fitness, given the elements of such a state. Both are needed to approach your potentials for wellbeing and long life. There are common understandings of physical fitness, but less consensus about the nature of mental fitness, though the topic has been extensively explored.

It may be just semantics, but what other quality of mental fitness might we suggest that seems overlooked in the WPA definition?

We suggest a sense of contentment, a good deal of the time. Contentment means a state of being happy and satisfied, relatively free from worries and restlessness with ample experiences of peace and relaxation. Contentment is not a gift from the gods, a state found in just the right combination of medications or a capacity to stand on one's head while chanting a mantra. Achieving contentment follows a pattern of mental conditioning, comparable to the physical fitness level derived from months of training in a pool, on a bike and/or running/walking regularly.

Of course, the mental fitness state of contentment, even in the face of a sea of troubles large and small, is invaluable at all stages of life. If you have not practiced calming techniques so far, consider your advance toward seniority status as a fine time to get started.

Consider these tips:

- Prepare for an increase of disappointments with age - the aches and ailments, unwelcome changes in society, noisy children, doctors who dispense bad news and so on. Exercise your contentment muscles so that week by

115

week, month after month, you find yourself better able to bear heavier loads of potential disturbances with less expenditures of worry, alarm, fear or dismay.

- Resolve to increase your mental REAL wellness skill of contentment. This will safeguard your ability to reason, enjoy, move and feel as free as conditions allow.

- Try to interpret the beginning stage of all troubles, whether simple disappointments, pains or limitations, as challenges or alerts to refocus. All such troubles signal the need to protect your serenity, calm and resolve to smile and enjoy as much as possible.

Of course, contentment in this sense of mental fitness is not easy, nor is physical fitness now or during your earlier life—if this were so, nearly everyone would be in a state of optimal wellbeing - and we all know that's not the case.

Think of mental fitness, with contentment being the foundation of this splendid state of being at all ages, as a heroic act - and a gift to others with the good fortune to observe and learn from your modeling of successful aging.

Robert W. Goldfarb captured these sentiments in a recent essay in the *New York Times*:

If there is one characteristic common to friends who are aging with a graceful acceptance of life's assaults, it is contentment. Some with life-altering disabilities — my blind friend, another with two prosthetic legs — are more serene and complain less than those with minor ailments. They accept the uncertainties of old age without surrendering to them. A few have told me that the wisdom they've acquired over the years has made aging easier to navigate than the chaos of adolescence. (Source: Robert W. Goldfarb, *The Secret to Aging Well? Contentment.* The New York Times, October 2, 2018.)

40. EMPLOY ARTFUL DEFIANCE AND GRACEFUL DODGING

Some things are easy; successful aging is not among them. Growing old is filled with losses, large and small.

Aging successfully requires many acts of resistance, often against well-meaning pressures from family and friends to conform to old-person stereotypes and customs that may not fit with the way you want to live out your retirement years. We recommend defiance! That is, safeguard your freedoms with resistance and graceful dodging whenever society or customs hold out lower expectations or fewer hopes. Resist advice to take it easy. Older people who are fit and looking after themselves are underrated - they don't want to hear well-meaning advice not to overdo it. They enjoy overdoing it, that is, living beyond the normalcy of mediocrity that society expects of seniors.

While favoring free speech and all the other liberties we enjoy, Winston Allen offered an example of graceful dodging, which can be the better part of unnecessary or injudicious valor:

> *I learned a long time ago that, unless you are very familiar with a person or persons, it's usually wise to avoid commenting on sensitive subjects, like race, religion or politics. Nowadays you can add right-to-life issues, gun control and climate change. Comments on these issues can alienate a whole bunch of people. Life is too short for that. Don't go there!*

We noticed that Winston did not include comment on the topic of sex in that list. Supposedly, some things are just too important to ignore, no matter the risks.

Maintain a high standard of living strong, for as long as you can manage to do so. William Hazlett suggested *the art of life is to know how to enjoy a little and endure much*, though we want to enjoy much, as well.

As children, we were told to act our age! That meant stop behaving like a younger, immature child. Well, that was silly -

we were still immature and still acting our age. We were children. We had no choice. But, as seniors, we think the opposite advice makes sense - don't act your age! That is, resist stereotypical elder behavior. Our 75+ champions often mentioned the fact that they, too, are *off put* by peers who act old when doing so is optional, that is, while they have the capacity to think, behave and otherwise function with more dynamic vitality than they exhibit.

All the tips that our champion centennials have offered support staying young in action if not appearance. Vigor and attitude far outweigh chronological age in conveying a dynamic presence. Do your part to eliminate outdated images—perk up and be your best *bright-side-of-life* self.

This is not to suggest denial of altered realities, but rather to offer support for giving ground grudgingly - while remaining in good spirits. Do what you can to keep the last act played out on your terms. Graceful and strategic retreats are little works of living art.

41. STRESS IS JANUS-LIKE—EMBRACE THE POSITIVE SIDE

The two sides of stress are the positive and the negative. The word stress overwhelmingly is associated with the negative. Yet, the dual nature of stress has within it a freedom-enriching opportunity.

No one can eliminate negative stresses entirely (e.g., fear, disappointment, worry), but the more you seek out, embrace and consciously utilize positive stresses (e.g., training and competitions, vacations, cultural experiences), the less noticeable the downer variety will affect you.

Stress is generally understood as a state of mental or emotional strain or tension resulting from adverse or demanding circumstances. But this definition of stress defines a person's response to stress, not the event or circumstance that created the condition of strain or tension. We can't control all events or circumstances that affect us; we can manage our responses. Doing so involves a combination of mental awareness and calming skills, as well as interpretations of events and circumstances that lower negative emotional levels in the body and brain. Robert Service might have had this idea in mind when he counseled,

Be master of your petty annoyances and conserve your energies for the big, worthwhile things. It isn't the mountain ahead that wears you out—it's the grain of sand in your shoe.

Positive stresses represent welcome excitements in anticipation of good returns from emotional encounters of varied kinds. This is the good kind of stress, technically known as *eustress,* but a lot of the not-so-good variety—worry, fear and anger—should be minimized and avoided, as much as possible. The events and circumstances causing stress are inestimable—examples range from family dramas to technological complexities (e.g., user frustrations that vex the unwary non-tech, genius-impaired types)—but not grandchildren, who seem to know everything about computers and cell phones. Basically, we might do well enough if we simply relax and take things one step (or even two or three steps) at a time.

Fix the things you can and get a little help figuring out the rest.

Stress is affected by everything going on in your life. It will keep you on the defensive, less open to seeking new freedoms, new ways to experience excitement and satisfaction. If you are in a fully functioning, effective life situation, negative events will still be negative but less likely ruinous. If your capacity for managing change honed over time has been well developed, whatever happens will be addressed and a steady state will return.

42. AGING WELL IS UNCOMMON - BE EXCEPTIONAL

Liberate yourself - in addition to the personal benefits, you will be rendering a public service for all seniors.
The norms for aging are grim; the physical and mental changes are unwelcome. We are too aware of the disquieting aspects of long-term survival (i.e., diminished functioning, more illness, less optimism, diminished sociability and so on), too unaware of alternative possibilities.

Aging well involves mitigating and delaying the downside of growing old while inventing attractive endeavors, distractions and varied entertainments that keep disquiet at bay. Your journey through senior-hood will be a solo venture, no matter how extensive your social and family networks. Even Queen Elizabeth II is on a solo aging trip - everyone else, the adoring crowds, the grumbling critics and the indifferent, are not at the wheel of your journey. Advice and assistance can be helpful, when desired, but you set the pace, the direction and the choice of stops along the way. A key element of aging well is to act boldly, protect your choices and embrace your individuality.

43. DRESS ANY WAY THAT MEETS YOUR FANCY

At every stage of life, there's no shortage of folks only too happy to suggest that what you're wearing looks good, is stylish or, more often, dated and no longer in vogue. When you're retired and immersed in living well, being happy and deciding things for yourself, it's time to ignore such busybodies.

Like you, fashions have evolved, so some concession to modern style might be considered, except perhaps on special occasions (e.g., Halloween). But *considered* is not the same as followed or believed or taken as holy writ or otherwise superior to your own seasoned judgment. Remember, you are at a perennial time of life, and you are firm and resolute, uncompromising about being the sovereign of your own personal freedoms. How you choose to dress is part of your commitment to liberty.

To feel at least middle-aged if not swank and voguish as a frat boy or sorority girl, pay a modicum of attention to fashions. On the other hand, maybe you prefer what some might think appears rather fuddy-duddy, geezerish or out of touch.

However lovely some of your frippery and raiments might be, they are museum worthy in the 21st century — La Belle Epoque (the Beautiful Era) and the Gilded Age are over. The opulence and extravagant King Edward VII, the once elegant trendsetting Gibson Girl dazzle repertoire of Alice Roosevelt Longworth, simply won't do in this era for most occasions, like supermarket shopping. Save the outrageous for stately funerals, Inaugural Balls and the like.

Do update your wardrobe now and then. Upswept bouffant hairdos are no longer all the rage and besides, they are not needed to look independent, charming and suitably youthful in spirit and panache.

However, if your children or grandchildren are not impressed and supportive of your textile choices, don't be intimidated. Wear what you like. It's probably too late to get new children and grandchildren, so let them know this is your way of feeling contemporary. Politely hint that they must not discourage your dapper instincts. And consider second and third opinions - you are a free agent and much prefer to make your own choices in these matters. So, thank you very much, boys and girls, and now back off, if you please.

Pay attention to and seek out a few opinions about fashion trends, not necessarily age-appropriate, but somewhat in line with your own sense of style. You've developed plenty of ideas about what looks good on you over the years. Keep this fashion sense in mind and be proud of it - it's part of who you are. Just don't be shy about getting regular fashion upgrades -

there are dances and concerts and such to attend, and you always want to catch the eye of folks who might be out there looking for a hot dude or a stunning babe with advanced life experience. Be alert to cultural forces that stereotype, overlook and under-expect older people. Adopt a personal dress code - and check your dapperness daily with a full-length mirror. To some extent, you feel how you look. Favor articles of clothing that make you feel sharp, fit, zestful and truly fine. Consider fashion tips from others, especially your mate, best friends and children - but you be the final arbiter.

Basically, you feel most confident when you look your best. Enforce an anti-old person dress code consistent with your budget. And don't forget that regular exercise is a vital part of fitting into a wardrobe that helps you look good. A fit body is the ultimate fashion statement at any age.

44. FAVOR LIBERATED COMPANIONS

People who treasure their own rights and prerogatives are the companions who will most respect and reinforce your own devotion to personal freedom.

For starters, don't hang out exclusively with old people. We have nothing against them—and we're certainly not prejudiced, since all of us are or hope to become old people.

But we need new blood to keep the vital arteries of social dynamism flowing unimpeded.

This is not as outrageously ageist as it might first appear. Mix it up with multiple generations, that is, go out of your way, if necessary (which it almost surely will be), to interact socially and otherwise with the young as well as with your peers and all the in-betweens.

All parties benefit from perspectives life impresses upon people at different time periods. Each age cohort has quite varied experiences going through the stages of life, such as high school and college, entry into the job market, marriage and so on in markedly different eras. Consider the prevailing cultures the 18 participants featured in this book knew in the 1940s. Imagine how modern teens, if time-travelled en masse into the 40s and 50s, would react to the norms of that era.

Countless forces, some easily recognized but most not even consciously assessed, shape the lives of generations once or twice removed from each other. It's only natural that different generations have impressions that vary about almost everything, given the evolution of society from the mid-20th century to the present time. With open minds, curiosity and good listening skills, old and young will have much to share and, hopefully, with which to entertain each other.

Sharon Roggenbuck captured this spirit with this observation:

Younger generations not only seem more liberated but also strike me as more outgoing and happy. Most of my friends are much younger, some younger than my own kids. Yet, we seem to relate well, enjoy each other and share happy outlooks. So, it's a fair, even serendipitous exchange, I think. In any case, they keep me young and I help them appreciate the fact that being old is no big deal.

Inspired perhaps by free-spirited Maude (Ruth Gordon) in the classic movie *Harold and Maude,* I think elder women ought to consider taking a male youth under their wings in a mentor (femtor) capacity. It won't work as well in reverse, due to unfortunate suspicions likely to arise. Besides, young men are in greater need of sensible guidance than their female counterparts.

45. ATTITUDES ARE HUGE - REFRESH REGULARLY

We sink or swim, prosper or languish, rise or fall with our attitudes and opinions. For the most part, we inherit both. We are the heirs of attitudes, habits and mental customs. (Ingersoll)

Negative attitudes or, more accurately, the lack of positive attitudes that attract, welcome and benefit others while harboring good feelings within, are inimical for thriving and flourishing. Experiment now and then by re-assessing certain attitudes, especially those held for a long time, passed along initially as traditional ways of thinking and embraced without deliberation during your earliest years. Your life is very different now from how things were then, including society, family and cultural influences that shaped your thinking and predispositions, for better or worse. Negative attitudes often take form over time, like the buildup of cholesterol in coronary arteries, and you know where that will lead.

A Stanford Research Institute study a few years ago estimated that success is 88% related to attitude relative to the rest, attributed to education. This was not meant to denigrate education but rather to highlight the power of attitudes, particularly those unconsciously adopted.

Almost all of us have been urged to change our attitude, initially by parents and teachers, later by coaches, bosses, military drill instructors and yes, even spouses. It's a good idea to consider such advice and make adjustments when appropriate, particularly when doing so enables added success at living well, that is, healthfully and happily. Change, whether of a situation under your control or not, is seldom easy. You might need to work on the change for a long period of time or, if beyond your influence, professional help may be necessary. Nothing shameful about that - the only shameful thing is to ignore a problem and thereby lose precious time for life enjoyments.

Bottom line - liberate yourself from tired, ineffective attitudes that no longer reflect the real you, should any such mental relics persist.

46. PRACTICE FORGIVENESS BUT GET IT RIGHT

If you can't forgive and forget, pick one. Forgiveness does not change the past, but it does enlarge the future. Paul Boese

One of the popular holy books suggests that a god promised to forgive those who would forgive others, but there are additional reasons to do so, with plausible benefits here on Earth. By forgiving, you don't allow your mind to fill with negativity. Forgiveness is the right thing to do because it is the better and nobler way to get on with anger-free functioning. As Ingersoll noted in a letter written on July 1, 1897, forgiving is a good idea simply because *no man can afford to make his heart a den of vipers.* (Source: *The Letters of Robert Green Ingersoll,* collected and edited by Eva Ingersoll Wakefield.) It's easy for a god to forgive enemies, since nobody can harm a god; for mere mortals, forgiveness can sometimes be *a big ask* - a formidable challenge. This is the case if you believe the hurts inflicted were severe. Yet, absent forgiveness, there are likely to be lasting feelings of anger, resentment, bitterness and maybe even thoughts of vengeance.

Forgiveness might also lead to reconciliation and/or possibly greater understanding, empathy and compassion. All these returns contribute to physical, emotional and mental wellbeing. Forgiveness does not require or necessarily entail forgetting, excusing or making up with whoever inflicted harm. Forgiveness is instead a choice to promote a level of peace that facilitates getting on with life, leaving anger behind.

Roger Little weighed in on this matter, pondering the nuances of the tip:

> *At first take, it seems an unmitigated good thing to make amends, or otherwise revisit a relationship, incident or situation that does not feel right, many years after occurrence. We all have unresolved issues of one kind or another with others. If things don't feel right, why not seek some peace, closure, warmth and/or the like?*
>
> *An unexpected call after a long period of silence risks catching the ex-wife or other estranged party either unprepared or just at a bad time. How about a letter? This allows a review of circumstances extant at the time of the break, a summary of your latest reflections, an affirmation of*

the good feelings and affections and the invitation to resolve matters. But, don't let your expectations get out of hand - it might be too much to hope for a reunion that lets the good times roll, as in the halcyon days of old.

If you are still not convinced to forgive that &$*^%$@ who did you wrong, consider this: *To forgive is to set a prisoner free and discover that the prisoner was you* (Louis B. Smedes), or this from Oscar Wilde, my own favorite: *Always forgive your enemies - nothing annoys them so much.*

Bottom line—forgiving can be liberating.

On the other hand, let's be real. Not everyone can forgive. You may be one you can't. You may prefer to hold a grudge. If you're going to do that, be good at it, in a way that does not pull you down, causing unnecessary, unpleasant vexation.

Aristotle's ethics featured a doctrine of the mean, wherein virtues and vices are found on a continuum and the right way to act is artfully between ineffective, incorrect extremes. In the case of forgiveness and anger, Aristotle would have us seek the right amount of anger for the right reason, at the right time, toward the right person.

There is a book that will tutor you in this skill - Sophie Hannah's *How to Hold A Grudge*. Ms. Hannah believes,

131

reasonably enough, that not everyone can forgive and move on, free as the birds in the sky. The world, after all, is filled with absolute wankers, so just try to let it go at that.

47. YOU RAISED YOUR KIDS, LET THEM RAISE THEIRS

Enjoy the grandchildren but don't live with or supervise them. If finances, family stability and other factors do not require a rescue intervention by caring and able grandparents, back off and give your children ample space to parent their clan. Provide grown children with the opportunity to raise their little darlins with the loving skill and nurturing you afforded them when they were in your care during their formative years. Treat your occasional visits as celebrity guest appearances - and depart with the tots wanting more. Ideally, they should be overjoyed when you show up. Why? Because you're fun, non-bossy, interesting and a change of pace - so long as they act somewhat sensibly and appropriately, even for little people, on occasions.

It's true that being surrounded by family can be delightful, now and then (mostly then) but the adults need privacy, as do your children and grandchildren. If you find yourself alone late in life, explore options other than moving in with family. Favor housing situations that bring potential new friends - that's the way to go, if possible.

Bill Zeiring added another perspective to this tip:

> *As parents our responsibility was to teach our children right from wrong. Now many of us are grandparents - and we realize we learned a few things from them, as well. As little people, they seldom walked when they could run. They rarely gorged at the dinner table. Most were well proportioned, and they laughed and smiled a lot, probably more so than I recall doing when their age. They were color blind and cared not at all about the economic status of their friends.*

The baton has been passed to your children to do the teaching. Sit back and give them room—and enjoy the good times, while delegating the rest—you've done your part.

48. TIME IS OF THE ESSENCE - TREAT YOURSELF WELL

Some of the 56 tips are easier to implement than others; none is more difficult, for most readers, than this one. We introduce this tip with a couple hypothetical statements:

> What if you are diagnosed with a fatal condition, and additional tests and medical opinions confirm that only a miracle will save you? What goal or goals would you have for the time remaining?

To stimulate your thinking about an action plan in the event of this dire occurrence, assume that you remain able-bodied and capable of getting around to do the things that matter to you. Now what? How would you live in the most positive ways to make the most of time available?

As the tip title indicates, we recommend in such a case that you treat yourself generously, doing things that will bring as much joy and meaning, fulfillment and more as possible. In fact, we recommend it for everyone in his or her later years.

So why do we suggest that treating yourself well might be difficult, that this tip will be a struggle to adopt and implement for most people? It does not on the face of it sound hard, does it? What's the big deal that makes us think treating ourselves well is not *a piece of cake, a cakewalk* or *easy as pie?* Because for most, doing so will go against the grain, will seem selfish and too little focused on the feelings, needs, priorities and expectations of loved ones. Your family and best friends, despite a world of good intentions, will act as to inadvertently focus too much attention on mourning, fears, doom and gloom, and too little on having one hell of a good time in the months you have remaining.

Therefore, we have a recommendation. We urge that you take steps to reassure all kind and loving folks, particularly family, that you appreciate them and respect their needs. However, and this is where you might encounter some difficulties, you have specific ideas for what you want to do, and being sad, worried or otherwise less than happy are not or will not be part of your action plans.

So, start thinking about what, if you are ever in this kind of situation, you might want to incorporate in your life that's new and different that will enhance positivity in living fully, even when the sands in the hourglass are running low.

Is it wise to wait until that reality becomes evident? Of course not. Commence at once to muse on actions to take if, someday, you find yourself in an overtime situation. By *overtime* we mean, to use a sports analogy, when the game is nearly over but you have an extra period in which to finish in style. That is, on the proverbial top of the mountain, thanks to the adroit usage of good calls, best plays, strategic timeouts and other ploys that enable what Ingersoll described as *sucking dry the orange of life,* leaving behind naught but the peelings.

To focus on your life at the final stage is not as self-centered as it might, at first, seem. Assume you made provisions affecting your heirs, business, causes and all the rest. After that, treating yourself well above all else comes down to this: How to experience the most happiness, joy, love and other qualities of exuberance in your remaining months?

135

We urge a conscious decision to do what it takes to enjoy life as much as possible, and as worry-free as you can manage. Focus upon your own desires, knowing you have devoted a lifetime of being exceptionally considerate of loved ones. No second guessing your choices from here on out! Get out there and do what still can be done. Spend some money! Your survivors will manage just fine. Seize the days to enjoy a few of life's little luxuries. Enjoying some of those resources you earned and conserved over a lifetime. No longer should you forego joys, adventures, the satisfactions of supporting favorite causes or other choices you desired but denied yourself in earlier times. Retire at last your deeply imbedded sense of frugality and responsibility for others. You've sacrificed long enough. You've harvested a modest fortune, perhaps. Do something, many things - for yourself with this little treasure chest.

Beware of televangelists, insurance salespeople and others who want to help - in return, of course, for your financial support for their special interests. Some may have legitimate products or services, a few may prove beneficial, depending upon your circumstances. However, don't overlook the fact that a merchant's overarching interest is his or her own interests. Get second opinions on possibilities as to proven quality and performance.

This is your last opportunity to live fully, to enjoy one thing or another or many things you may have long pondered. Go ahead and indulge long-delayed possible delights. Yes, consider but don't be constrained about the financial situation of children or grandchildren—or their future children and grandchildren. Eschew any guilt about spending on yourself. You've taken care of loved ones for years and, in doing so, provided a fine head start. At last, your turn has arrived. You have nurtured, educated, sheltered and otherwise provided a good deal of support for a very long time. Perhaps it's time to turn a bit of generosity your way. Who would object?

Wouldn't it be odd, and a bit mental, if each generation scrimped and saved, went without for their children and grandchildren, who then kept the cycle going ad infinitum, generation after generation? Nobody would get to live fully, take enough holidays, experience special things and events or otherwise enjoy the fruits of their labors, since all would feel compelled, obligated or guilted into saving for the next line of future sufferers in the bloodline.

There would be no end to the cycle of frugality and sacrifice. Quite irrational. Liberate yourself. Time is of the essence. Jack Welber offered this take on this matter of deriving maximum consequence at the end of one's days:

For me personally, the strongest argument for going positive is one that focuses on leaving a positive legacy for family and friends. My overarching goal is to provide an example that contains a mix of courage, enlightened self-interest and attendant details involved in death.

Give yourself a proper send off.

49. LIVE WELL AND DIE HEALTHY

Do this for your sake and as a generous and wise legacy for family, friends and generations to come.

Most of us expect to leave a modest legacy to our descendants, though few are in a hurry to do so. There's no point in rushing this form of generosity. Consider this: You are shaping your legacy now. Why not take added steps to create a legacy of having lived well and fully, particularly during your senior years? Why not, when your physical self has returned to stardust, be remembered for having aged successfully? Yes, the atoms and molecules and every cell that comprises the being that is you will eventually reoccupy infinitely small parts of our expanding and amazing universe. The universe is, after all, a boundless immensity of millions of billions of galaxies, each with billions of stars, incomprehensible in its massive grandeur. If you have not traveled widely so far in life, no worries—when you're done here, your 37.2 trillion cells (more or less, depending on body size) will get around like nobody's business.

As for religious ideas that posit a soul, well, in that case perhaps your non-material spirit will go somewhere else, for better or worse, depending on whether you had the right belief system and followed its doctrines sufficiently.

50. BE A PHILANTHROPIST IN YOUR OWN UNIQUE WAY

No act of kindness, no matter how small, is ever wasted.
Aesop

If lucky enough to have been born into wealth and/or other favorable circumstances, or having earned such through your dedicated efforts, consider redirecting some of your resources, talents and energies to liberate others from want. Assisting others to enjoy a few of the personal freedoms you have come to appreciate will surely prove satisfying.

No doubt you can think of many attractive possibilities, such as supporting policies and programs that improve the prospects that babies are wanted and born with healthy minds and bodies. Similar ideas might include promoting science education or working to bring about a more effective secular democracy that equally guarantees freedom of and from religion, in accord with individual choices freely made.

Simple acts of kindness, such as visiting the infirm in order to cheer up one or more elders whose conditions do not provide much in the way of social interactions, varied experiences and the like would be a most generous form of philanthropy.

Viktor Frankl, Irvin Yalom and other existentialists insisted that the surest roads to happiness were to be found along paths of service to others. Again, recalling the wisdom of Ingersoll, he suggested that *Improved Man would find his greatest joy in the happiness of others...and he will reap his greatest reward in being loved by those whose lives he has enriched.*

51. YOU ARE NEVER TOO OLD TO ENJOY SEX

Well, at some point you might be, but go out of your way now to explore possibilities before it's too late.

Healthy sexuality, consensual and safe, legal and harmful to no one, is a natural and splendid way to celebrate your freedom and good fortune. Moderate expectations, but don't abandon your interests in a healthy sex life. Very few will encourage it, most will disapprove of it and nobody will admit to it. Do it anyway - a perennial has as much right to a sex life as anyone else.

Sharon Roggenbuck suggested that *being in love can make you look and feel younger. Having lost the first love of my life I was*

fortunate to find another man to love. He has brought me much
pleasure and happiness. My friends say I absolutely glow with
happiness and vitality.

Unfortunately, while desire comes easily and naturally,
execution is complicated by certain realities. Unless you have
something like Dr. Emmett L. Brown's truly cool DeLorean
equipped with a time travel accessory like a *flux capacitor* to
transport you back about 30 years for some hot action, you
must moderate your expectations.

One of the realities to accept and to which you must adapt is
that certain things have changed. Today, you are probably not
quite as drop-dead gorgeous as you were 30 years ago.
Furthermore, you are no longer a stellar athlete or the student
body president, the playboy stud/homecoming queen of a
prestigious university or the heroine in the school musical,
idolized as if you were the King or Queen of England.

People are so shallow. Why should any of this make you less
adorable? Good luck.

52. FREE SPEECH IS YOUR BIRTHRIGHT - EXERCISE IT LIBERALLY

No need any more to be politically correct, to fret about blasphemy or to otherwise refrain from giving offense to the easily offended.

This, of course, is not the case if you happen to live or otherwise find yourself in countries like Pakistan, Saudi Arabia, Iran, Russia or any of the totalitarian, theocratic or other authoritarian nations whose leaders are implacably hostile to freedoms enshrined in our Bill of Rights, Declaration of Independence and Constitution. Despite a long history of leaders seemingly given to a few totalitarian, theocratic or other authoritarian tendencies of their own, we continue to benefit from the wisdom of our Founders and the conviction of leaders who now and over time have taken our birthright liberties seriously.

It's important to be sensitive, attuned to the feelings of others, tolerant, kind and reasonable rather than cranky and difficult. That does not mean you can't harbor and even express controversial views on any topic that meets your fancy, even if your opinions are out of the mainstream and likely to offend some. After all, this is America and so far, it's still legal to be outspoken, even a little outrageous.

Many folks nowadays really are quick to take offense. This predisposition will conflict with your First Amendment rights. Americans take pride in free speech. Since the 15th of December 1791, Congress has been on notice by our Constitution to

> *make no law abridging the freedom of speech.* Article 1 of the Bill of Rights also forbids constraints *respecting an establishment of religion or prohibiting the free exercise thereof; or of the press; or the right of the people peaceably to assemble and to petition the Government for a redress of grievances.*

So, speak your mind when so inclined and, if someone doesn't like it, well, that's just too bad. Here are three examples of potentially non-PC tips for successful aging:

1. Stay away from crowds—other people are generally unattractive, noisy, rather daft and carriers of mostly morose attitudes, superstitions and contagions.

2. Keep to the front of the train as Jim Jefferies advises— *That is where all the scientists and intelligent people ride, forging the way forward for the rest of humanity. It is only a small, select group of mostly non-conformists making it possible for the throngs in the trailing cars to manage at all.*

3. Be rich and hire many servants. Have you noticed how most of the members of royal families live long and happy lives, like for example the Queen of England? Doing nothing for yourself takes away the daily stress of living. No need for exercise—follow this rule and your private chef can prepare healthy and delicious meals three times a day. When money is no object, people pay to come and stare at your opulence, as they do today at George Vanderbilt's 8,000-acre estate in the Blue Ridge Mountains of Asheville, NC and William Randolph Hearst's grand castle on a hilltop in San Simeon, CA. All this and additional self-indulgences will leave you feeling superior and extraordinarily more worthy than the commoners. As an old tongue-in-cheek proverb goes, *if the rich could hire other people to die for them, the poor could make a wonderful living.*

We're kidding. You're not likely to have any interest in hiring servants or building castles. The freedoms you enjoy enable all the little pleasures that make life worthwhile and delightfully pleasant.

53. FOCUS ON THE BIG PICTURE

Transcend surviving - that's essential but pursue a higher standard, namely, to flourish and thrive.

The important thing is the present. No incident, misstep or other setback from the past need be tolerated as a weight on your mind or a drag on your optimism. Adopt that philosophy and regrets will soon diminish into the proverbial ash heap of your history. Recall the previous reference to the Python *Galaxy Song*, which further described the bigger picture of our planet, our galaxy and the universe evolving, revolving, orbiting, moving, going round and expanding at speeds over distances that are unimaginable and simply gobsmacking. This will help you lighten up—your birth was amazing and unlikely in the first place, so make the best of being along for the ride around our sun at 19 miles a second. That is, so it's reckoned.

54. PRACTICE YOUR CONVERSATIONAL SKILLS

The alternative, which has widespread appeal, is inadvertently becoming a gasbag jabberer.

Tune up your conversational skills or, if you haven't any, familiarize yourself with the fundamentals. Consider this five-word formula for being an effective conversationalist who liberates others to speak freely: *Talk less and listen more.*

You probably know people who barely give others a chance to get a word in and, when they do, interrupt before the other can finish a sentence. Can you think of anyone like that?

Here's a hint: Watch a talk show, such as *Hardball* with Chris Matthews on MSNBC. It's an informative show with excellent guests, but the moderator can be insufferable. He often asks a panelist a question but offers his answer to the query before the exasperated panelist can get a word in. Sometimes, Matthews allows a few moments for a reply, but rarely does a guest get to finish before being interrupted. So, another way to suggest that you become a skilled conversationalist is watch *Hardball* - and resolve not to be like Chris Matthews.

55. BE AS STOIC AS YOU CAN MANAGE

> *You have power over your mind - not outside events. Realize this, and you will find strength.* Marcus Aurelius, *Meditations*

A stoic is a person who can endure pain or hardship without whining, moaning or groaning incessantly. Zeno of Citium founded the Hellenistic philosophy called stoicism in Athens during the early 3rd century BCE. Stoicism, an early form of liberation from anxiety and distress, flourished throughout the Roman and Greek world until the 3rd century CE. To last that long, there had to be something to it, a functional advantage throughout life, especially during the later years when there was so much more to whine, moan and/or groan about.

Stoicism entails the endurance of pain or hardship without a display of feelings, with patience, forbearance, resignation, fortitude, endurance, acceptance and tolerance. Stoics are largely indifferent to the vicissitudes of fortune. Some schools of stoicism go too far - they also promote the dreadful idea of being indifferent to happiness or pleasure. We are strongly opposed to this aberrant aspect of stoicism. We are enthusiastic supporters of happiness and pleasure, provided such is not at the expense of another. As Ingersoll observed,

> *No one should fail to pick up every jewel of joy that can be found in his path. Everyone should be as happy as he can, provided he is not happy at the expense of another, and no person rightly constituted can be happy at the expense of another.*

Of course, as with other worthy disciplines, stoicism about pain and discomfort does not come naturally or without earnest efforts. What's more, it can be overdone. If you trip and fall or suffer any kind of setback or pain, you're entitled to a good gripe and a brief excursion into self-pity, now and then. The key is to get over it - and return to your normal state of serene poise and elegant grace. All manners of dysfunction are part and parcel of getting older.

Ingersoll noted the following:

> *Arguments cannot be answered with insults...kindness is*
> *strength...anger blows out the lamp of the mind. In the*
> *examination of a great and important question, everyone*
> *should be serene, slow-paced and calm.*

This tip is not meant to deny arguments, anger, pain and suffering, but rather to discourage excessive attention to such tribulations. This is best for the sufferer, as well as those suffering the sufferer. Physical and other difficulties are a part of the cycle of life. To the extent possible, resist granting much attention to discomforts - seek out distractions and diversions from troubles. Cultivate the mind; become *familiar with the mighty thoughts that genius has expressed* as distractions and diversions. Arthur Schopenhauer advocated the alleviation of suffering through an appreciation of aesthetics, altruism and asceticism. Ingersoll, author of the above phrase about *mighty thoughts,* would add love and hope to the remedy, believing as he did that *love is the only bow on life's dark cloud,* and *hope is the consolation of the world.*

Admittedly, this advice is easy to give, but grief and suffering endure and require time to moderate. In such cases, a foundation philosophy such as stoicism for mental calm can be invaluable. To the extent possible, view difficulties as something nearly all mortals experience and, despite it all, strive to recapture your usual tough, resilient, capable and positive state as soon as possible.

56. LIBERATE YOURSELF

Be vigilant about safeguarding your personal freedoms as the years go by. Developing and putting to use a strong capacity to live on your own terms is not only a right and a privilege of modern life in progressive societies, but a duty to yourself and others who rely on your good judgment. Investigate for yourself the questions, problems and mysteries of life. Take notice of widely held beliefs of majorities of people, but only as a guide or starting point. Keep in mind that no established falsehood is popular enough to bribe your judgment or still your conscience. You don't have to convince others to see things your way in order to make the best choices based upon how you want to live.

Kenneth Fleischhacker advised against allowing beliefs to harden, to become somewhat ironclad. He illuminated the suggestion with a revealing tale as to how he came to embrace this notion:

> *One of my old work acquaintances, who was suspicious of my 'clean-living nature boy' lifestyle, offered me and fellow co-workers a celebratory cigar after his wife had a baby. I accepted, and to be non-controversial, I even smoked it (gag),*

as did others in our group. I think the gesture not only changed his attitude towards me, which had been a bit standoffish, but also sparked a bit of an epiphany about the healthy lifestyle types, to the point that, albeit in a limited way, he started to model his behavior after my own.

As Ingersoll noted: *I am doing what little I can to hasten the day when the human race will enjoy liberty, not just of body but liberty of mind, and by liberty of mind I mean freedom from superstition, and added to that, the intelligence to find out the conditions of happiness, and added to that, the wisdom to live in accordance with those conditions.*

Epilogue

First and foremost, Don and Jack thank their 16 world champion friends and competitors for their time and wisdom in providing the material for this book. The year-long process had many thrills and a very sad moment. To our deep dismay, one of our own, Elizabeth Brackett, lost her life doing what she thoroughly enjoyed — training for a triathlon.

So, let us suck this orange of life dry, so that when death does come, we can politely say to him, you are welcome to peelings. What little there was we have enjoyed. Robert G. Ingersoll

Postscript

The extensive research and interviews that led to the production of *Not Dead Yet* took place over a one-year period. Eligible participants were identified by USAT. Champions 75+ who had won one or more world titles were invited to participate. Nearly all agreed; a few who declined did so for health or privacy reasons. We thought all eligible triathletes had been contacted, but we missed one distinguished champion, namely, Wayne Fong, of Los Angeles, a six-time world champion born in 1932.

When we produce a second edition, perhaps after the sale of the first million or so copies, you can be certain that the redoubtable Wayne Fong will be featured, along with Wayne Fong stories and other insights he will surely contribute.

Chapter Six

Biographies

DON ARDELL, CO-AUTHOR

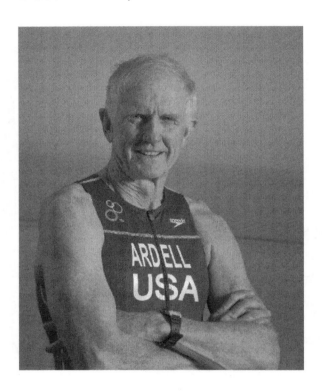

Don has authored 15 books, including *High Level Wellness: An Alternative to Doctors, Drugs and Disease* (Rodale, Bantam and Ten Speed published separate editions between 1977 and 1988). This book was the impetus for the wellness movement that exists today. In presentations throughout the U.S., Canada, Europe, Australia and Asia since 1977, Don has focused on positive, enjoyable ways to live better via exuberant living. He has specialized in assisting organizations transition into effective, rational cultures that support positive lifestyles.

Don has degrees from The George Washington University, The University of North Carolina (Chapel Hill), Stanford University and The Union Institute and University (Cincinnati). He is the recipient of lifetime achievement awards from the Global Wellness Institute, the National Wellness Institute, the German Wellness Institute and the Japan Wellness Institute. He was one of 10 Americans to receive the Healthy America Fitness Leaders Award in 1993 from the President's Council on Physical Fitness and Sports, Allstate Insurance Company and the U.S. Jaycees. He is an All-American triathlete and duathlete and has won over a dozen national titles and seven world championships (in Tasmania, Montreal, London, Edmonton, Budapest and the Gold Coast of Australia). He is the current national champion in both triathlon (Cleveland) and duathlon (Greenville, S.C.).

Don writes the Ardell Wellness Report (860 editions to date since 1984), lectures on REAL wellness, the life and speeches of American orator Robert Green Ingersoll (1833-1899) and promotes his patent for a 2-step/no hands/no bending heel design for fast triathlon transitions.

JACK WELBER, CO-AUTHOR

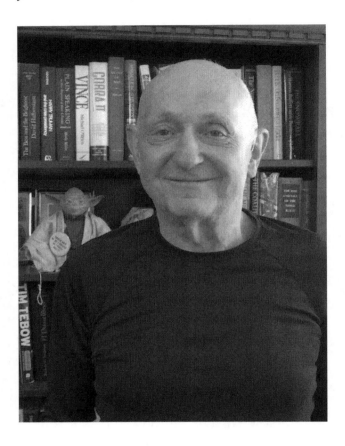

Jack graduated from the University of Florida in Gainesville with a BA in economics and a minor in philosophy in 1959. He then entered military service with the U.S. Army, where he became a specialist 4th class chosen as a piccolo and flute player in the 24th Infantry Division Band. Jack was recruited by Johnson & Johnson in 1965, where he spent 27 years in various middle and senior management-level positions. He also performed as the first flutist in the Doctor Symphony Orchestra in New York City from 1964 through 1966, and as a flutist for the Greenwich Village Woodwind Quartet. After early retirement in 1992, a second career was enjoyed in the pharmaceutical industry as a physician recruiter.

Eventually (2004), Jack formed his own recruiting firm. This endeavor proved very successful, as his Wimbledon Group placed over 50 physicians, mostly oncologists, at Bristol Myers Squibb, Johnson & Johnson, Pfizer and other companies. In recent years, Jack has enjoyed publishing short stories, essays and family histories.

A lifelong athlete, Jack was a member of his high school basketball and track teams. He began doing triathlons in 2005 and reached the podium in ITU world triathlon events in Penticton, Gold Coast and Rotterdam (gold medal winner in 2017).

Jack plays bridge, occasionally online chess and recently took up meditation, using an app created by Sam Harris. He is developing an online character self-assessment that explores the nine traits described by David Brooks in *The Road to Character.*

JON ADAMSON

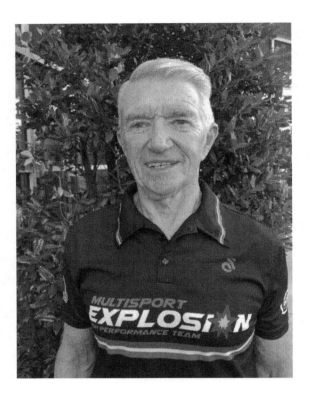

Jon was born January 5, 1937 in Racine, WI where he spent his elementary and high school years. He played basketball and football in junior high, but his size (5'8" on a 150 pound frame) did not encourage continuing with either sport at the high school level. He noted, it was too bad there was no cross-country team option - I was pretty fast and might have done well.

Jon served in the U.S. Marine Corps for two years after graduation, after which he enrolled at Marquette University where he earned a degree in mechanical engineering. He played some club tennis and racquetball during his prime working years, but it was pretty much all work, not so much play. In 1978, he returned to college, graduating in two years with an MBA from Vanderbilt.

At about this time, he decided to invest more energy in health and fitness. He took up running and, lo and behold, discovered he was pretty good at it. In most local races, he found himself on podiums - and before long developed an appetite for higher places on those podiums. As serendipity would have it, he and his running buddies discovered a new sport, triathlon!

Jon's first tri was a positive experience and he was hooked. Soon thereafter, longer races and greater challenges beckoned. He did the first of his four Boston marathons in 1984.

Jon attributes his good results to genetics, a strong work ethic, a favorable environment, positive attitudes and perseverance. He recommends giving back what wisdom you've discovered and applied.

Jon coaches athletes young and old and encourages them to pursue their dreams. While he gets paid for coaching, he points out that it is definitely not work.

WINSTON ALLEN

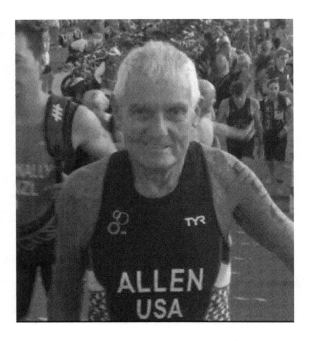

Winston was born April 13, 1930 and brought up in Columbus, OH.

Winston's interest in exercise commenced at age nine when he realized he was smaller in stature than his peers, and thus might have to defend against school bullies. Among other initiatives, Winston joined a YMCA and learned to swim. To earn the coveted title *minnow*, he had to swim the length of the pool. After he finished the qualifying lap, the instructor said, *Hey kid, you're good*. That was, as the song goes, the start of something new. In due time, Winston became a formidable swimmer in high school and college and, in later life, in the first leg of triathlons. Funny how a few words, on occasions, can affect a life.

As a swimmer and diver, initially at Ohio State University, he decided early on that he might be a small fish in a big pond. Thus, he transferred to DePaul University in Chicago, where it was the other way around - he was now a big fish in a small pond. However, at DePaul, Winston won a national diving title, suggesting that he was, in fact, an impressive fish in any pond, large or small.

A retired military officer, Winston served in both the US Air Force and the US. Army. While in the Air Force he was an OSI (Office of Special Investigations) special agent. He was also the first springboard diving coach at the Air Force Academy. Later, he studied to become a Japanese linguist, graduating from the Defense Language Institute at The Presidio in Monterey, CA.

Winston retired after a 22-year career as a U.S. Army officer.

Winston's strategy for triathlon competitions is, *if you can't beat 'em, outlive 'em!*, while adding, *I have enjoyed many successes, none possible without the help of others.*

DAVID ARST

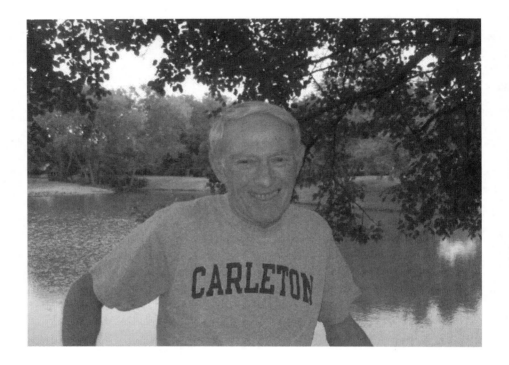

David was born August 2, 1933 in Wichita, KS where he grew up and remains today.

As he describes it, growing up was wonderful. His folks doted on him and his brother, spoiling them both in good ways. David played baseball with neighbors in a lot at the end of the block and basketball in his driveway. Alas, this routine was the high point of his early athletic years.

In high school, he took up smoking and drinking. By the time he showed up at Carleton College in Northfield, MN, he did not appear to be the most physically gifted young man on campus. After graduating, he enrolled in law school at Kansas University. His career was set in motion. He's still practicing law full time.

David had bypass surgery in 2003; shortly thereafter, a friend suggested he try triathlons. He was 70 years old and wondered if people take up such sports at 70. He'd have to learn to swim, re-learn how to bike and run well enough to enjoy the effort and do well in the age group.

A decade later, after many triathlons, things came together for David in an epic experience in Edmonton, Canada. In the 2014 World Triathlon Championship, David won the Sprint Triathlon title. He has a favorite memory from that occasion, which he described as follows:

As I made the final turn to run past the grandstand, the announcer called my name as the new world champion in the 80-84 age group.

This was an almost indescribable 'one moment in time'. I so wish everyone could experience something like it. Never forget: each of us is a champion in one way or another.

ELIZABETH BRACKETT (1941-2018)

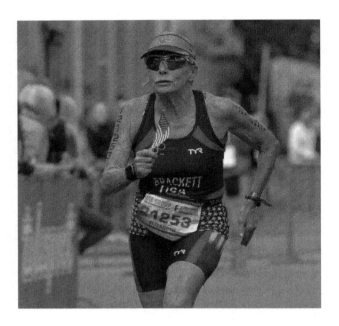

Elizabeth was born December 11, 1941 in Minneapolis, MN. A longtime Chicago journalist, she died June 17, 2018, four days after a fall while riding her bicycle along the city's lakefront training for an upcoming triathlon.

Elizabeth attended the University of Wisconsin-Madison but transferred to the University of Indiana to maximize her diving talents. She was the first woman on the University swim team. As a journalist and reporter, Elizabeth became an Emmy-winning host for *Chicago Tonight*. She covered many national events, such as political conventions and scandals, pro basketball and many disasters, among other local and national stories.

Elizabeth was a full participant in the writing of this book. When asked about dealing with frailties, finding meaning and the value of competing in later life, she offered the following:

Discovering triathlon at age 50 changed my life. It gave me the discipline I needed to get back into shape and to set realistic, achievable goals. I watched the bodies of my contemporaries weaken while I was getting stronger. I had not found a way to stop the aging process, but by getting into the best possible shape, I slowed that process—a lot.

I've become a little more realistic about my eventual demise. I occasionally lift the layers of denial and peer into the future. I know there will be a time when my body will let me down, a time when swimming, biking, running and maybe even walking will no longer be possible. I don't know what would be worse—losing my physical abilities and having the mental capacity to know it or losing my mind while my body remains strong. Given my years of training, it's likely to be the latter.

Of course, neither sounds very appealing. Contemplating these unpleasant endings sends me back to my standby coping mechanism—denial. So far, it's working just fine.

ROGER L. BROCKENBROUGH

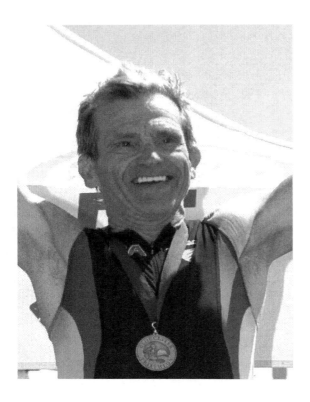

Roger was born July 31, 1934 in Buena Vista, VA. He attended Virginia Tech University in Blacksburg, VA, graduating with a BS in civil engineering, to which he added a master's in structural engineering. His career commenced as an officer in the Army Corp of Engineers, mostly at Fort Benning, GA on bridge-building and small construction projects, after which he spent 30 years with U.S. Steel's Tech Center. Roger took an early retirement at age 57, at which time he got serious about having more enjoyment in life! (However, due to the lingering effects of the Protestant ethic, he continued with part-time engineering work for another 30 years.)

Roger was inducted into the USA Triathlon Hall of Fame in 2017.

Roger continues to enjoy engineering work - at present he's updating a 5th edition of his technical opus, *Structural Steel Designer's Handbook,* a single source of the latest design codes, standards, specifications and other information essential to the practical design of steel structures.

MARGARET BOMBERG

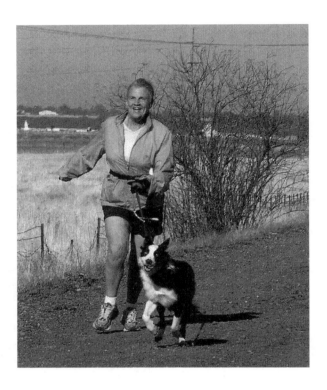

Margaret was born April 24, 1937 in Boston, MA. Her early years, however, were spent in Long Beach, CA.

While initially a teacher, her calling seemed destined to be in the legal profession. Margaret's mother went to Cornell Law School and her father to Harvard Law School. While only her father continued along the lawyer track, so did her husband and, eventually, Margaret as well.

In 1979 at age 42, Margaret moved to Chico, CA.

Margaret entertainingly elaborated on her belief that she possessed no special talents as an athlete in her youth. When classmates chose sides for kickball, field hockey and so on, whoever picked first got the right to assign Margaret to the other side. When that option was not respected, she was picked last. Margaret suggests her tale might suggest another approach to fun and glory in multi-sports quite different from others who exceled in athletics at an early age. For example, consider that persistence pays off, especially when others fail to show up. Margaret noted that most of the time only one or two in the very senior groups show up. Furthermore, as often as not, you're the only one. In that case, all you have to do is finish. Bring a flashlight, if necessary!

Margaret has five children and is thankful that their father was very athletic. Her three daughters were athletic when young and remain in competitive shape today. Her two adopted sons are also quite vigorous.

Margaret herself, despite the *aw shucks* downplaying of her innate talents, has competed in every national championship from 2006 to 2016, except in 2009. She also earned the right to compete as a member of Team USA in 12 world championships, winning gold medals in three of these events. She said, *Oh, I wish those girls who picked me last could see me now.*

Margaret still finds the training to be fun and the friendships to be priceless. She runs with a group and still takes swimming lessons, in part to ensure that she remains on top of the water in races.

SUSAN BRADLEY-COX

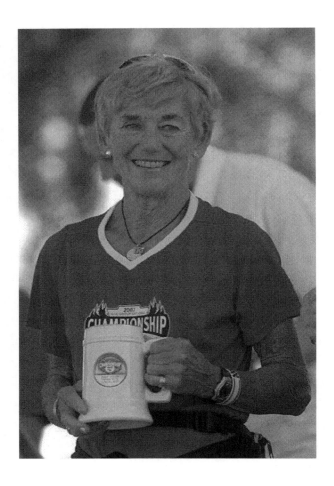

Susan was born November 9, 1937 in Paducah, KY. She grew up in a small town, an environment she describes as being wonderfully supportive. She enjoyed the college years at the University of Kentucky, seizing every opportunity to express gratitude to all who opened doors, offered opportunities and encouraged her to strive to be her best. There being no swim team for women at the time, Susan excelled in synchronized swimming and gymnastics. Susan's post-college career has focused on guidance counseling, managing outdoor programs, assisting adults with special challenges to experience sports, coaching cheerleading, masters-level swim teams and other water sports. She also assists a Team-in-Training group that raises funds for leukemia/lymphoma research.

An annual triathlon is held in Susan's name (*Tri for Sight* – a fundraiser for eye research at UK). Susan's motto is, *No one flourishes alone – be grateful to all for encouragement and for opening doors.*

Susan was inducted into the USA Triathlon Hall of Fame in 2010.

EILEEN CROISSANT

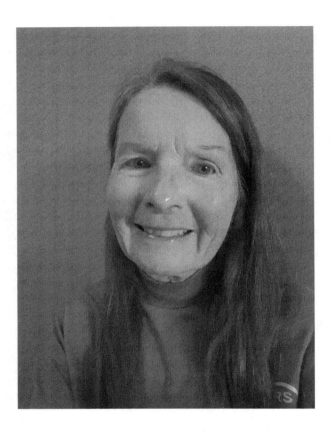

Eileen O'Hare was born in Beloit, WI on September 19, 1939. In that Dark Ages period of American sports culture, females did not have much opportunity to enjoy sporting activities with their peers - most popular sports were deemed unladylike. Girls were cheerleaders (a sport that's more demanding than it looks). As a child, Eileen learned to swim, though of course there were no female swim teams or even practice opportunities.

Eileen eventually moved to Colorado, got married, had four children and didn't think about swimming until her late 30's when her kids were on swim teams. This led Eileen back to the pool, swimming laps along with the parents of swimmers. She also joined a fitness center in order to swim year-round.

Eileen and her husband also biked a good bit, at least until he shifted his focus to running, as did many of her friends. Though she went to races, it was years before she decided to give running races a try. One friend was training for a triathlon - Eileen hadn't heard of triathlon. When her health club organized one, she volunteered to help. Soon enough, Eileen decided *I can do that*. A year later, at age 48, she did her first triathlon, finishing not last, but close to last. That didn't matter - she was hooked.

Eileen did not consider herself an athlete growing up, though it's unlikely she doubts that now after winning her age group (75-79) at the World Triathlon Championship in Chicago in 2015.

Eileen was a chief financial officer for several community health clinics and found it necessary to cut back on competitions during a 15- year career, though she continued to exercise. When she turned 70 and began part-time work, she decided it was time to return to triathlon training.

KENNETH FLEISCHHACKER

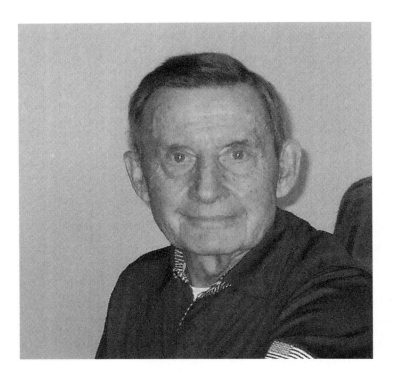

Ken was born April 30, 1936 in Chicago, IL. He was active in multiple sports while living in one of Chicago's many ethnic enclaves. He enrolled at Wilbur Wright College, later transferring to Loyola University of Chicago where he majored in exercise physiology. His early career commenced at Western Electric, followed by a stint of military service with the U.S. Army in Germany. Ken took up badminton while there, winning several military championships in both singles and doubles. Returning to Western Electric after discharge, he eventually relocated to Denver, CO where he got to indulge his love of skiing. Before retiring early, he led company wellness programs. Ken is convinced that successful aging is not a solo journey.

As to special interests that focus his attention during the later years, Ken offered quite a tale. It seems he devotes considerable time to genealogy, long a matter of interest, given a combination of family lore about European immigrant ancestors and a capability of digging deep with computer software. In addition, Ken's spouse is steeped in genealogy, so the investigatory database has been growing for years.

Here's what Ken said about this avocation:

> *One story I discovered concerns my Austrian grandfather, a railroad worker. On one fabled occasion, he had to pursue a runaway train! After a considerable distance, he caught up with the last car and managed to stop the unsupervised progression, a heroic act for which he was no doubt feted and, we hope, promoted. In doing so, passenger and other lives were saved. As the story goes, he died shortly thereafter, presumably in part due to the emotions and rigors of this incident. While this sounds like the basis of many cowboy movies, it also tells me where some of my endurance genes may have come from. I'm still on a quest to verify if this folklore is at least partially true.*

PAT FOSSUM

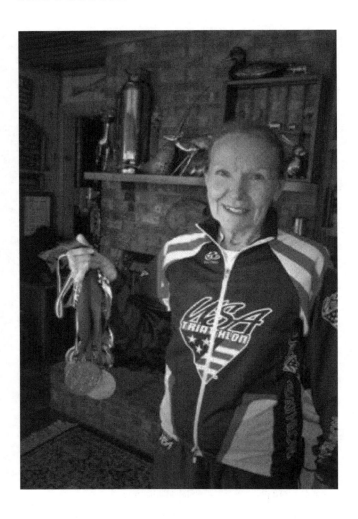

Pat was born February 18, 1935 in Albert Lea, MN where she grew up loving the ice and snow. She earned a BS in education from Macalester College in St. Paul and later a master's degree from Auburn University in Montgomery, AL. She married her high school sweetheart, an Air Force officer and travelled the world, teaching at each new assignment. Upon retirement, she continued her active lifestyle in Montgomery. After battling two major health problems, breast cancer and stroke, she resumed training, as doing so is conducive to her desire to set and achieve goals. Pat believes it is never too late to start – *start slow and go!*

Pat and husband Jerry devote most of their time to the challenging quest to obtain and sell highly selective fine antiques, often maintaining as many as five booths at malls and exhibitions.

BRUCE HILDRETH

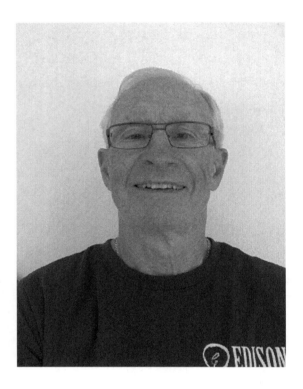

Bruce was born April 21, 1940 in Iowa. He started duathlon training at age four, riding his bike everywhere around his hometown of Ames, Iowa. He participated in all sports as a youth but didn't excel. He attended Iowa State University, followed by med school, also at Iowa State University. After military service, he commenced his medical career in California. A good part of his career was in the Lake Tahoe area as an emergency physician where his free time was spent snow skiing and mountain biking.

Bruce retired in 2000, bought a boat and lived aboard in the eastern Caribbean for five years. Tiring of the sedentary cruising life, he sold the boat in 2005 and moved to a land-based tropical life in SE Florida, where staying fit was much easier. While competing in an adventure triathlon, he met his future wife, a runner. She encouraged him to start running seriously at age 65. This resulted in both winning division titles in running races, duathlons and triathlons. Medical issues arose at age 68, leading Bruce to observe, perhaps not originally, that aging takes a toll. It seems the best athlete in the most senior groups is frequently the one who stays the healthiest. Bruce suggests that one of the best ways to age successfully is to be of service to others.

ROGER LITTLE

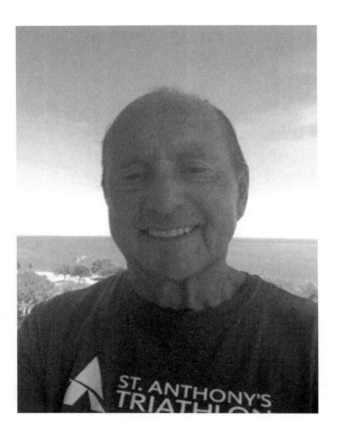

Roger was born September 28, 1940 in Adams, MA, a small town in the Berkshire Hills. Growing up, he was active in baseball, football and basketball. Roger first attended Colgate University, after which he earned a master's at MIT in geophysics. He has lived most of his life in Bedford, MA but now spends winters in St. Petersburg, FL. From MIT, he started at an engineering company. Over nearly half a century he created new companies in the solar, semiconductor, biotech and defense industries.

Roger attributes the tenacity, determination and perseverance required for success at triathlons as qualities of value in a business career. He believes that living well and staying in shape is the best way to live and eventually the way to cross the finish line of life.

At present, Roger serves as the chief technical officer of a company called N2 Biomedical that he spun off from another firm he started and sold. N2 Biomedical, whose CEO is Roger's son, is developing a marijuana breathalyzer.

DWIGHT LUNDELL

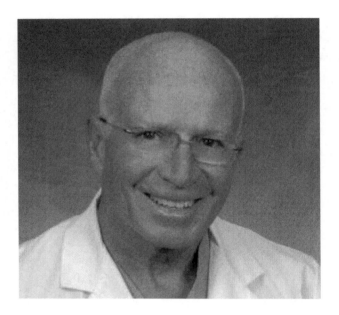

Dwight was born November 23, 1943 in Safford, AZ. He attended the University of Arizona as an undergraduate, after which he was selected to the charter class at the university's college of medicine where he completed general surgery training. Next was a residency in cardiovascular surgery at Yale University. Dwight returned to Arizona and built a successful cardiovascular practice. During his career, he performed over 5,000 coronary bypass procedures and countless valve, thoracic and vascular operations.

Dwight does not consider himself a natural athlete, just a determined one. In his view, determination trumps talent;

success derives more from persistent effort than anything else. Despite the difficulties, injuries and pains, he considers himself well compensated for investments in late-life athletics. In his estimation, older folks, contrary to popular myths, still have goals and aspirations, things to accomplish, experiences to enjoy.

Currently, Dwight consults with and formulates products for nutrition companies, is completing a second book and continues to enjoy Ironman training.

SHARON ROGGENBUCK

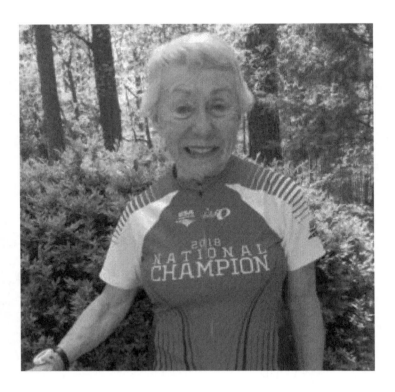

Sharon was born October 20,1938 in Peoria, IL. A good share of her youth in Peoria was spent caring for and riding horses. She attended college for one year at Bradley University, followed by a year and a half stint studying dental hygiene at Marquette University. Sharon's education was put on hold by marriage and raising four children. After the family moved to Michigan, she was able to complete her dental hygiene degree and soon after a bachelor's degree in health science at Western Michigan University. Ten years of work in this field followed. At age 40, Sharon became an athlete, competing in running races, duathlons and triathlons, competing at the local, national and world level. For 30 years she has been doing two-day cycle rides raising funds for MS related research. Currently, Sharon teaches exercise classes to pay for her races. She also is part of a tap group that performs in shows and at nursing and retirement homes.

LOCKETT E. WOOD

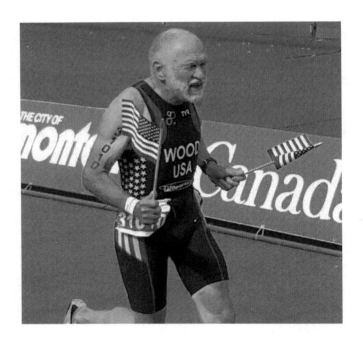

Lockett was born August 1, 1939 in Albuquerque, NM. While he was active in sports as a youth, including playing football and running track in high school (not very good, he noted), he ran his first triathlon at age 70. He obtained degrees in physics and electrical engineering from the University of New Mexico. He also did graduate work at Brown University and the University of Colorado, where he obtained a Master of Science and a Ph.D. in electrical engineering. Highlights of his career at Avivid Technologies Group include positions as CEO, marketing VP, senior scientific manager and chief scientist. He founded several startup technology companies.

One of his companies (Colorado MEDTech) ultimately employed over 500 engineers and technical support people. Dr. Wood holds 33 patents and has published 30 scientific papers.

One under-appreciated benefit of growing older as a triathlete/duathlete comes every five years – moving into a new age group. This is one of the few things all triathletes eagerly anticipate about growing older – Lockett suggests it might in itself be reason enough to take up multi-sports!

Lockett continues working full-time and enjoying every day this side of the grass. At 73, he started yet another company capable of purifying industrial waters. As he explained,

> *My wife doesn't understand why I don't want to go on vacations. It's simple - I'm doing important work that excites. I am on vacation, every day. This keeps me energized and I feel better today on the cusp of 80 than I did at 37 when I was overweight.*

BILL ZIERING

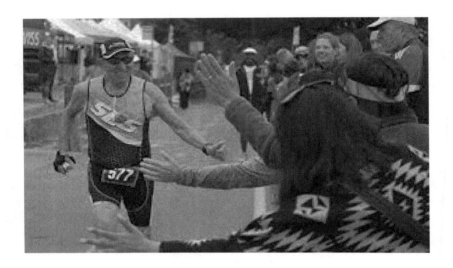

Bill was born January 22, 1930 in New York City and grew up in four of the city's five boroughs. He enjoyed playing every game on offer, though he reports excelling in none. Bill graduated from Michigan State University, then obtained a master's degree at the University of Michigan and followed that with medical school at Northwestern. He interned in Brooklyn and then went to live in Chicago during a residency at Northwestern Children's Memorial Hospital. He served in the Marine Corps for a few years before returning to Chicago for further medical training. Many posts later in various California cities, he settled down in the Central Valley. Bill incorporated wellness principles in his professional practice, at an early time, well before doing so became popular.

Bill has been the world champion in his 85-89 year-age-group since 2015 and plans to be in Lausanne this year to make it a clean sweep. Of interest is the fact that *Pokey Bill,* as he calls himself, didn't learn to swim until his mid-50s. Over the last six decades he's completed 40 races. What's his secret? *It's just perseverance and discipline and finding a few secret thrills in life.*

For the past dozen years, Bill and his wife Pam have run a ministry, *For The Least Of Us,* funding needy families in crisis.

Appendix

List of Tips by Page Numbers

Reason Dimension   Tips   1 – 13   Pages 23 - 52
Exuberance Dimension   Tips 14 – 24   Pages 53 - 74
Athleticism Dimension   Tips 25 – 36   Pages 75 - 108
Liberty Dimension   Tips 37 – 56   Pages 109 - 150

REASON DIMENSION

1. Choose A Life of Disciplined Excellence
2. Wellbeing Requires a Highly Fit Brain
3. If You Are Aging Well, Share Your Tips
4. Danger - Hazmat Alert on the Use and Disposition of Pills
5. Be Optimistic - Perhaps All is for the Best, but Verify
6. Appreciate Being Alive Now, During the 21st Century
7. Seek Companions Who are Rational
8. Curb Your Enthusiasm for Medical Miracles
9. Whenever Life Gets You Down, Think Big
10. Mute the Ads
11. High-Risk, Low-Return Initiatives—Forget About Them
12. Surgeries: To Be or Not to Be (Operated On)
13. Surgery as a Gamble

EXUBERANCE DIMENSION

14. Go Out of Your Way for Humor, Fun, Joy and Happiness

15. Be Adventuresome

16. Be Bold, Spontaneous and Gregarious

17. Let Charming and Likable Be Your Personality Homepage

18. Influence and Dazzle

19. Give Homage to Marcel Proust - Remember Friends Past

20. Be Grateful

21. Ponder the Possibilities

22. What a Specimen Thou Art!

23. Have Something Special on the Horizon

24. Perform a Good-Humored Secular Exorcism

ATHLETICISM DIMENSION

25. All Tips are Equal but This One's More Equal

26. Don't Call It Quits Too Soon

27. Eat Well

28. Is It Too Late?

29. Join A Well-Equipped Club

30. Treat Yourself to Regular Massages

31. Get It Done, But Don't Be Tyrannical About It

32. Choose A Favorite Diet

33. Explore Some Form of Meditation

34. Slow Down, Be Calm, Chew Thoroughly

35. Stand Tall, Chin Up, Keep Your Shoulders Back

36. Know the Facts and Trends of Aging

Liberty Dimension

37. Extend to All the Rights You Claim for Yourself

38. Complaining Is Mental Junkfood - Find Alternatives

39. Contentment - The Mental Equivalent of Fitness

40. Employ Artful Defiance and Graceful Dodging

41. Stress Is Janus-Like - Embrace the Positive Side

42. Aging Well Is Uncommon - Be Exceptional

43. Dress Any Way That Meets Your Fancy

44. Favor Liberated Companions

45. Attitudes Are Huge - Refresh Regularly

46. Practice Forgiveness but Get It Right

47. You Raised Your Kids, Let Them Raise Theirs

48. Time Is of The Essence - Treat Yourself Well

49. Live Well and Die Healthy

50. Be A Philanthropist in Your Own Unique Way

51. You Are Never Too Old to Enjoy Sex

52. Free Speech Is Your Birthright - Exercise It Liberally

53. Focus on the Big Picture

54. Practice Your Conversational Skills

55. Be as Stoic as You Can Manage

56. Liberate Yourself

Acknowledgements

We appreciate the support extended since Day One by:

- Tim Yount and Lauren Rios of USA Triathlon, the governing body of our sport
- Wellness pioneer John W. Travis, M.D. and Bill Dunn, the Editor Emeritus of the Freedom from Religion Foundation, for assistance editing the first editions
- Philip and Rachel Welber for technical and marketing advice in creating our Facebook page
- James Lafferty and Audrey Welber Lafferty for design and support with the Google Drive used for organizing and making data accessible for all our participants, for the graphics of the Grim Reaper chasing the co-authors (see back cover), as well as for our *NotDeadYetthebook* website and the Kindle edition
- Lloyd Botway - the mellow maestro most mellifluous for providing the voice for the *Not Dead Yet* audio book
- Our spouses, Carol and Emelia, for continuous encouragement, draft reviews, ideas, tolerance and patience.

To all we will remain somewhat eternally grateful; a few of the above will probably be remembered in our wills.

Recommended Readings Related to the Tips

Armstrong, Sue. *Borrowed Time: The Science of How and Why We Age*. Sigma, 2019,

Browne, Harry. *How I Found Freedom in an Unfree World*. Liam Works/Avon, 1973.

Cohen, Gene. *The Mature Mind: The Positive Power of the Aging Brain*. Basic Books, 2006

C.P. Farrell, *The Ghosts and Other Lectures by Robert Green Ingersoll*. New York, C. P. Farrell, 1892

Crowley, Chris and Lodge, Henry S. *Younger Next Year*. Workman Publishing, 2007.

Flynn, Tom and Roger E. Greeley. *Robert Green Ingersoll. In Tom Flynn, Ed. The New Encyclopedia of Unbelief*. Amherst, New York: Prometheus Books, 2007.

Fry, Prem and Keyes, Corey. *New Frontiers in Resilient Aging: Life Strengths and Wellbeing in Later Years*. Cambridge University Press, 2010.

Gawande, Atul. *Being Mortal: Illness, Medicine and What Matters in the End*. Picadore Press, 2015.

Greeley, Roger E., Ed. *Ingersoll: Immortal Infidel.* Buffalo, New York: Prometheus Books, 1977.

Gurian, Michael. *The Wonder of Aging: New Approach to Embracing Life after 50.* Simon and Shuster, 2013.

Handford, Thomas W. *Ingersollia: Gems of Thought from the Lectures, Speeches and Conversations of Col. Robert G. Ingersoll.* Gutenberg ebook.

Harari, Yuval Noah. *Sapiens: A Brief History of Mankind. Harper Perennial*, 2015.

Ingersoll, Robert G. *The Works of Robert G. Ingersoll.* 12 vols. New York: Dresden, 1900.

Jacoby, Susan. *The Great Agnostic: Robert Ingersoll and American Freethought.* New Haven and London: Yale University Press, 2013.

Larson, Orvin. *American Infidel: Robert G. Ingersoll.* 2nd Ed. New York: Citadel Press, 1992.

Middleton, Marc. *Rock Stars of Aging - Retirement Comm: 50 Ways to Live to 100 - Lifestyle Secrets of Centenarians.* Bolder Press, 2017.

Rauch, Jonathan. *The Happiness Curve : Why Life Gets Better After 50*. Bloomsbury Publishing, 2018.

Sagan, Carl. *The Demon-Haunted World: Science as a Candle in the Dark*. Random House, 1995.

Smith, Frank. *Robert G. Ingersoll: A Life*. Buffalo, New York: Prometheus Books, 1990.

VanTine, Julia. *Ageless Brain: Think Faster, Remember More, and Stay Sharper by Lowering Your Brain Age*. Rodale Press, 2018.

=============

(A note on the recommended readings. Several books are not focused either on aging or wellness. For example, we suggest seven books about Robert G. Ingersoll, because of our fondness for his memorable expressions related to the tips. Three other works, by Carl Sagan, Harry Browne and Yuval Noah Harari are included because they offer invaluable wisdom on three of the four themes of *Not Dead Yet* - reason, liberty and flourishing, respectively.)

The End

Made in the USA
Coppell, TX
08 June 2021

57057985R00107